THE HEALTH GUIDE TO

PMS

When you're faced with a pressing health issue, your first instinct is to find out as much about it as you can. With so much conflicting information out there, where can you turn for professional, supportive advice?

Packed with the most recent, up-to-date data, THE HEALTH GUIDES help ensure that you get a good diagnosis, choose the best doctor, and find the right medical treatment. With this one comprehensive resource, you and your family members have all the information you could possibly need—at your fingertips.

Accessible and easy to read, THE HEALTH GUIDES provide specific details and clear examples that relate to your given medical situation. If you're looking for one-stop, all-inclusive guides that allow you to understand and become more in tune with your body, this groundbreaking series is the perfect tool for you.

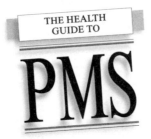

THE HEALTH
GUIDE TO

PMS

Dear Reader,

Just like many of you, for a long time I never thought about PMS and never even realized I might have it. I didn't pay attention to my periods, and because I was in overall good health, I dismissed any aches and pains as a minor interference. If I got irritated or upset, I blamed other things in my life—stress, work, a few too many dishes in the sink. If I gained weight, it was because I ate a few too many cookies and didn't exercise.

Then one day, I mentioned to my husband that someone I knew had PMS. "I'm glad I don't have it," I said. "Yes, you do," he replied. I was about to deny it when it hit me—he was right. It dawned on me just how many times I got outrageously mad and how often I was moody for no apparent reason. A few mental calculations later, I realized this happened around my period, when, eerily, I also seemed to gain weight. How could it be that I was an adult and just learning something so critical about my body?

Researching PMS and talking to many women who have it showed me just how complex PMS is, the extensive role brain chemicals play, and the large variety of strategies I could try to make myself feel better.

It's my hope that *The Health Guide to PMS* not only teaches you some things you didn't know about premenstrual syndrome, but that it convinces you that you don't have to live with PMS.

Best wishes,

Dagmara Scalise

THE HEALTH GUIDE TO

PMS

The essential guide to reducing discomfort, minimising symptoms, and feeling your best

DAGMARA SCALISE

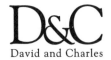

David and Charles

To Steve, Katrina, Hope and Julian,
for sympathizing and working hard with me.

A DAVID & CHARLES BOOK
Updates and amendments copyright © David & Charles Limited 2007
Copyright © 2007 F+W Publications Inc.

David & Charles is an F+W Publications Inc. company
4700 East Galbraith Road
Cincinnati, OH 45236

First published in the UK in 2007
First published in the USA as The Everything® Guide to PMS,
by Adams Media in 2007

A catalogue record for this book is available from the British Library.

ISBN-13: 978-0-7153-2817-0
ISBN-10: 0-7153-2817-4

Printed in Great Britain by CPD Wales
for David & Charles
Brunel House, Newton Abbot, Devon

Visit our website at www.davidandcharles.co.uk

David & Charles books are available from all good bookshops;
alternatively you can contact our Orderline on 0870 9908222 or
write to us at FREEPOST EX2 110, D&C Direct, Newton Abbot,
TQ12 4ZZ (no stamp required UK only).

The recipes in this book are reprinted with permission from F+W Publications,
Inc.; the United Soy Board; Recipezaar.com; The No-Salt Cookbook by David C.
Anderson and Thomas D. Anderson, copyright © 2001 by F+W Publications, Inc.;
The Everything® Low-Fat, High-Flavor Cookbook by Lisa Shaw, copyright © 1998 by
F+W Publications, Inc.

Acknowledgments

I'd like to thank Kerry Smith; Gina Panettieri; recipe authors Lisa Shaw, David C. Anderson, and Thomas D. Anderson; the folks at Talksoy.com and Recipezaar.com; Melissa Maehl, Mary Rawlins, Holly Duncan, Laura Engel, and Deborah Cousino; Barbara Novosel, Jane Jeffries, Claire Lillis, and Susan Rizzo; my mom, Krystyna Dobrzynski; Beverly and Rose Scalise; and last, but certainly not least, Julian, Hope, Katrina, and Steven Scalise.

Contents

Introduction

Premenstrual syndrome is well known but little understood, both by the women who have it and the physicians who treat them. At times, it seems that every woman around has PMS, but it never looks the same. One woman swears she's bloated and craves chocolate; another has crying fits and mood swings, while a third gains weight or has insomnia. The symptoms range all over the map. What's worse, you can't do anything about it, right?

Even though it affects 80 percent of women, PMS can't seem to get any respect. In fact, our culture loves to make jokes about PMS and how it makes women lose control. There's nothing funnier or scarier than a woman who gets enraged because there's no ice cream in the house, or because her husband forgets to do something he was supposed to do.

The jokes exist in part because there are a lot of misconceptions about PMS and its causes. Some people think it's just a normal part of a woman's life while others refuse to believe it exists. Neither of these opinions are true, however. PMS is confounding: it includes more than 150 symptoms that happen to occur during the menstrual cycle. This complexity makes PMS difficult to identify and to treat. It also provides the perfect opportunity for people and businesses to crowd the marketplace and hawk purported PMS cures, such as the many dubious therapies that abound on the Internet.

Medical experts haven't deciphered all of the mechanisms involved in PMS, but they do know it is driven to some degree by brain chemistry. The neurotransmitter serotonin seems to play a central role. PMS is also driven by a woman's family history, her diet, and her lifestyle. On a biological level, some women are simply more predisposed to getting PMS. It may be a relief to many sufferers to know that there are valid medical explanations for those infamous mood swings, anxiety, and irritability—there's even a biological explanation for PMS food cravings! For the small percentage of women who have severe PMS, it is a relief to know that their devastating symptoms are part of a legitimate disorder rather than something they're imagining.

Though our culture considers PMS a "female thing," premenstrual syndrome affects more people than the women who have it. It takes its toll on a woman's family, on her relationships, and even on her job. Researchers recently calculated that PMS costs society billions of dollars as each woman diagnosed with PMS accrues more than $4,000 in direct and indirect costs, such as days lost from work, lost productivity while on the job, and medication costs!

Unfortunately, many women simply give up in the face of such a diffuse disorder: they're confused by their symptoms and wonder what, if anything, they can do about them. PMS treatments vary from simple at-home strategies, such as taking pain relievers and adjusting how you eat and exercise, to hormone treatments, antidepressants, and numerous alternative therapies; navigating through them can be tricky. *The Health Guide to PMS* tries to provide answers to your questions about what PMS is, what it isn't, and what you can do about it.

The truth is that women with PMS don't have to give up and accept their symptoms as a matter of course. *The Health Guide to PMS* is a comprehensive resource to help you beat it.

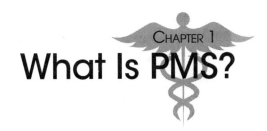

CHAPTER 1

What Is PMS?

PREMENSTRUAL SYNDROME, COMMONLY KNOWN as PMS, afflicts as many as 55 million women, making them irritable, achy, depressed, and anxious. According to the American College of Obstetricians and Gynecologists, at least 85 percent of women with regular menstrual cycles have at least one PMS symptom. Unfortunately, just because PMS is common doesn't mean it is well understood, and that puts women with PMS at a disadvantage: they may not know what is bothering them or how to get help. They think they're forced to live with their symptoms. What's worse, women with PMS are too often ridiculed or dismissed, when all they really want is relief.

Is It a Myth?

Because PMS is poorly understood, it may be easy to write it off as a myth. Not every woman gets PMS symptoms, and the symptoms themselves come and go in cycles. The range of symptoms is also very broad. For every woman who is irritable or anxious, there is another who is bloated, suffers headaches or backaches, is depressed, or has trouble sleeping. The intensity of symptoms can vary from woman to woman or from month to month. This variety and complexity can make self-diagnosis difficult.

It is also true that many women don't understand their bodies or their menstrual cycles very well and so have difficulty recognizing and understanding that they may have PMS. Additionally, many women insist they don't have PMS, while their husbands, boyfriends, or partners insist they do.

A woman who is feeling irritable may be genuinely upset or affected by something; she may be stressed by work, school, or her home life; or she simply may have had a hard day. She may also be experiencing PMS. It's difficult for her to pinpoint what is going on unless she actively pays regular attention to her body and her emotional state; she needs to have a reference point that enables her to distinguish when she is feeling normal or "off."

PMS symptoms can also be confused with symptoms of other physical illnesses and mental disorders. As a result, those women seeking treatment may be misdiagnosed, treated for conditions they don't have, or not treated for conditions they do have.

Sometimes what appears to be PMS is actually a different illness or condition. Depending on the particular constellation of symptoms, the condition could be one of the following:

- Hypothyroidism
- Irritable bowel syndrome
- Depression
- Pelvic inflammation
- Premenstrual dysphoric disorder
- Seasonal affective disorder
- Dysmenorrhea

Types of Myths

There are persistent cultural misconceptions about PMS. One myth, as illustrated in the earlier section, is that PMS makes women overly emotional, even deranged. These types of portrayals, so common in popular culture, rarely include the physical symptoms of PMS, such as joint pain, breast tenderness and swelling, or backache. Women who are "PMS-ing" are just more intensely emotional than women who are not, the myth suggests.

Another misconception is that women use PMS as an excuse to behave badly: to feel angry, to be upset, or even to go off their diets! In this view, PMS is seen as a convenient excuse that allows women to "get away" with something.

There's even an argument that PMS is, itself, a myth. For example, Australian scholar Jane Ussher believes that PMS is used by medical professionals to cover up the unhappiness women experience from modern-day life and the pressure to be superwomen. "PMS [is] essentially a form of repressed rage women feel rather than a medical illness," she writes in her 2006 book, *Managing the Monstrous Feminine: Regulating the Reproductive Body.*

Another myth about PMS is that there is nothing a woman can do about it; she must suffer through it as best she can. This idea is damaging because it prevents women from seeking and getting genuine relief from PMS symptoms. It is even more damaging to the small percentage of women whose very severe symptoms interfere with their everyday lives. The truth is, there are a number of strategies and medications that can help alleviate PMS symptoms.

Common PMS myths include the following:

- PMS turns women into emotional wrecks.
- PMS is an excuse to behave badly.
- PMS is not real.
- PMS is normal for all women.
- A woman can't do anything about PMS.

What Is the Reality?

Premenstrual syndrome is a real condition, with specific, identifiable symptoms, and it has been around for a long time. The medical community first recognized PMS in 1931, more than seventy-five years ago, but there have been descriptions of the disorder since ancient Greece.

Symptoms

PMS symptoms fall into three categories: physical, emotional, and psychological/behavioral. These symptoms tend to worsen in the one or two weeks prior to a woman's period and then disappear by the end of a full menstrual flow. Common PMS symptoms include:

Physical
- Pelvic bloating
- Swelling of the hands or feet
- Breast tenderness and swelling
- Acne flare-ups
- Food cravings
- Headache
- Upset stomach
- Constipation
- Diarrhea
- Migraine
- Joint and muscle pain
- Fatigue or exhaustion

Emotional
- Moodiness
- Irritability and oversensitivity
- Anger or sadness
- Crying spells
- Tension
- Increased sexual desire

Psychological/Behavioral
- Anxiety
- Depression
- Social withdrawal
- Forgetfulness
- Difficulty concentrating/Fuzzy thinking
- Difficulty sleeping

Body and Mind?

While today the vast majority of health experts agree that PMS is real, it still remains a poorly understood condition. Experts are not certain of the specific causes, nor do they agree on the best treatments. Is PMS physical? Psychological? Or both? To what degree does lifestyle or heredity play into it? What about age or diet or hormones?

Since PMS was first identified as a medical condition in 1931, many experts in the medical community have questioned the premise that it is a "real" disorder. For a long time, many experts argued that patients simply imagined PMS. It wasn't until the mid-1980s that medical experts defined the criteria for a diagnosis of PMS. More recently, in the 1990s, researchers finally succeeded in convincing the medical community that an extreme version of PMS, called premenstrual dysphoric disorder, or PMDD, should be considered a mental health disorder with a biological cause. Even today, despite so much evidence to the contrary, there are some mental health experts who continue to remain skeptical about the validity of PMS and PMDD.

Essential

Just how many women get PMS? According to the American College of Obstetricians and Gynecologists, between 20 percent and 40 percent of women have symptoms significantly bothersome to qualify as PMS. Another 3 to 8 percent of women have the most severe form of PMS, known as premenstrual dysphoric disorder, or PMDD.

Part of the problem is that numerous illnesses exhibit PMS-like symptoms. Fatigue, common in PMS, may be the result of anemia, a potassium deficiency, or hypothyroidism; headaches may be caused by stress or, more seriously, by intracranial lesions; a gastrointestinal disorder may cause PMS-like bloating. The same problem exists for diagnosing PMDD, which may be confused with a panic or personality disorder. This is why medical professionals often have a difficult time diagnosing PMS and PMDD.

Discomfort or Disorder?

PMS affects women to varying degrees. For some, mild symptoms mean a monthly bout with discomfort that passes fairly quickly. For another 20 to 40 percent of women, PMS becomes a debilitating disorder that prevents them from participating in normal activities, such as work, exercise, or even interactions with their family. Of course, many women fall somewhere in the middle; their PMS is painful or disruptive enough that they seek relief from their symptoms, but not so severe that they can't function in their daily lives.

Consider this: Any woman who's stepped on a scale a few days before her period only to find she's gained a few pounds or who finds that her favorite jeans won't zip up because she's bloated has experienced PMS symptoms. As has the woman who finds she craves chocolate, potato chips or pretzels, or the woman whose skin breaks out, like clockwork, one week before her period is due. But these women may not think they have PMS; they're simply in a bit of discomfort.

There are many women with PMS who are lucky enough to experience only one or two mild symptoms. Maybe they get a little weepy watching a sad movie or are more tense than usual at work. Perhaps they get a slight headache or can't fall asleep as they normally do. Although these are all PMS symptoms, these women are able to get relief from over-the-counter painkillers, extra rest, or some exercise.

Others aren't so lucky. These women suffer through migraines that force them to lie down in a darkened room, or they literally can't get out of bed. They experience significant highs and lows: alternately moody or tense, angry or sad. Their emotional and physical symptoms are marked and severe. These women may be suffering from premenstrual dysphoric disorder. PMDD is a mood disorder that is distinct from normal PMS and should be treated by a medical professional. The doctor may prescribe a class of drugs called selective serotonin reuptake inhibitors, or SSRIs, such as fluoxetine (Prozac or Sarafem), sertraline (Zoloft), or paroxetine (Paxil).

How Common Is It?

A staggering number of women have PMS at some point in their lives. Recent studies show that up to 80 to 85 percent of women experience PMS symptoms, or about 43 million to 55 million women annually (based on U.S. Census figures). Between 20 and 40 percent of these women say the symptoms are bad enough that they cause a change in behavior that is noticeable by themselves and others. This group is considered to have "menstrual distress." A small number of women— between 3 and 5 percent—have PMDD, which is characterized by severe emotional and physical symptoms that affect their daily lives.

By definition, only women who are menstruating can get PMS. So girls and women who are not yet menstruating, menopausal women and women who are not ovulating—whether because they are pregnant or for some other reason—cannot get PMS because they don't have periods. Some experts have tried to divide PMS into different levels of severity:

- **PMS:** Low-level symptoms (mild discomfort), sometimes called premenstrual tension.
- **PMS:** Regular or standard symptoms, also known as menstrual distress.
- **PMDD:** Severe emotional and physical symptoms.
- **PMM:** Premenstrual magnification is not PMS but a condition in which other illnesses are intensified during the premenstrual phase.

Where you fall on the spectrum depends on the severity of your symptoms, but suffice it to say, whether you have mild or severe PMS, you are not alone.

The Official Diagnosis

Although a great number of women suffer from PMS, many aren't officially diagnosed. A medical diagnosis requires that a woman's social activities or work-related performance must be notably impaired and her symptoms must occur consistently during two cycles (and she must record or chart her symptoms). In addition, those symptoms must be unrelated to any prescription drugs or hormone therapies, or to drug or alcohol use.

 Fact

> The American College of Obstetricians and Gynecologists defines PMS as the cyclic occurrence of symptoms that are sufficiently severe to interfere with some aspects of life, and that appear with consistent and predictable relationship to a woman's menstrual flow, known as menses.

A 1999 survey of 445 U.S. women showed that nearly one-third (31 percent) of those reporting PMS symptoms met the medical criteria for PMS and that fewer than half (45 percent) with severe medical symptoms sought help. A staggering 58 percent did not think any treatment would help!

What Can You Do?

Contrary to popular belief, you don't have to be at the mercy of your symptoms. You *can* treat PMS. Some of the easiest strategies involve self-treatment; that is, altering your diet, committing to exercise, and changing your lifestyle. For some women, over-the-counter medications such as ibuprofen may provide all the relief they need; others may need more powerful prescription drugs. There are also dietary supplements, such as calcium or magnesium that have shown promise in relieving symptoms such as bloating, breast tenderness, mood-related symptoms, and migraine headaches. Some (though not all) women find that oral contraceptives can relieve their symptoms. (Chapter 18 discusses oral contraceptives as a PMS therapy in more detail.)

Alert

More than 300 remedies have been prescribed for PMS, including estrogen, oral contraceptives, diuretics, antidepressants, nutritional therapies such as vitamin B6 and evening primrose oil, surgery, psychotherapy, and even light therapy!

If your symptoms are more severe, you may want to contact an expert who can help diagnose and treat your PMS. However, here your choices are wide-ranging. Since PMS consists of so many different types of symptoms, the "expert" label means different things: physician, psychologist, counselor, or psychiatrist. Each specialist has different treatment plans or approaches. In addition, some nutritionists, dietitians, and practitioners of alternative medicine also consider themselves experts on natural PMS treatments.

Essential

There are multiple strategies to treating PMS: self-treatment, over-the-counter and prescription drugs, and alternative therapies, including chiropractic, reflexology, aromatherapy, and yoga. These strategies have different levels of acceptance among health-care professionals.

PMS in the Media

Ask the average person—male or female—to describe a woman with PMS, and you're likely to hear terms such as *irrational, disturbed, emotional, enraged, crazy,* and *cranky*—and those are just the clean terms! Those who don't have PMS either consider it funny or scary, and sometimes both.

The emotional mood swings that supposedly characterize PMS are often parodied in the media. On television and in the movies, women with PMS are alternately weepy or crazy, gorging on potato chips or chocolate, and in general, baffling the men around them with unpredictable behavior.

PMS on TV

These representations are not accurate, but they're usually played for laughs. Television sitcoms are a good example. In the last thirty years, numerous television shows, from *All in the Family* in the 1970s to *Everybody Loves Raymond* in the twenty-first century, have made fun of the emotional turmoil caused by women with PMS.

In 1990, the television show *Roseanne* aired an episode called "PMS, I Love You," in which Roseanne Conner, the main character, drives her entire family crazy because of her PMS. Her husband describes her PMS as being like a "24-hour roller coaster ride with Sybil at the switch."

More recently, Raymond, the lead character on *Everybody Loves Raymond*, proposes tape-recording his wife's PMS-induced rampages so she can hear how irrational and antagonistic she's being.

Here's a thirty-year history of TV sitcoms and PMS:

- **1973:** *All in the Family*—PMS pushes Gloria to yell at her mother, Edith, in an episode called "The Battle of the Month."
- **1983:** *Taxi*—In the episode "Simka's Monthlies," Simka, the Eastern European wife of cabdriver Latka, goes berserk; fellow cabby Elaine explains to the men that she has premenstrual syndrome.
- **1988:** *Married with Children*—Peg and Kelly Bundy and neighbor Marcy get PMS simultaneously on a camping trip. They growl, snarl, and demand chocolate; they scare the men so badly that the men prefer to face a bear that has trapped them in a cabin rather than face the women.

- **1990:** *Roseanne*—Roseanne drives her family crazy when she's PMS-ing.
- **2000:** *Everybody Loves Raymond*—Debra rages and complains there's no medication for PMS that can relieve all of her symptoms.

⌐ Essential

Even bumper stickers poke fun at the irrationality and supposed violence of PMS. Common messages on bumper stickers include:
- PMS = Punish Men Severely
- Watch Out! PMS Behind the Wheel
- I Have PMS and a Handgun. Any Questions?
- A Woman with PMS and ESP is a Bitch Who Knows Everything

The media finds it convenient and funny to write off a woman's anger as PMS. It gives the woman a reason to kick butt, seek revenge, and let her emotions fly. It also gives the male characters an opportunity to admit they'll never understand women.

Rhea Parsons, assistant professor of psychology at Borough of Manhattan Community College of the City University of New York, has analyzed images of PMS on television, including the *Raymond* episode. She argues that although these portrayals are meant to be funny, this kind of misrepresentation is harmful to women because it leads to the development of inaccurate ideas about the reality of PMS. "PMS is not portrayed as a women's illness," she writes in her article, *The Portrayal of PMS on Television Sitcoms*, "so much as an inconvenience to men…Perhaps the biggest change is that current characters on television actually say 'PMS' whereas thirty years ago, it was 'understood' by the women's 'irrational' behavior."

Fact

PMS has been used as a defense in the courtroom. Shoplifting charges were dropped against a Canadian woman when medical evidence showed that she had suffered from PMS since she was a teenager. Around this same time, a British barmaid was charged with murdering a coworker. Her defense claimed that PMS was a mitigating factor, and she was found guilty of manslaughter rather than murder.

Next Steps

For the women who suffer from PMS, it is far from funny. In reality, living through the symptoms month after month can be frightening. The first step is to learn all you can about your health and your PMS symptoms. Are your symptoms consistent from month to month? Are they related to any other issues in your life, such as work-related stress or other illnesses? How debilitating are they? This will help you choose a course of action. Understanding PMS starts with knowing all about your body and your menstrual cycle.

CHAPTER 2

The Menstrual Cycle

ALTHOUGH A WOMAN WILL get her period about 450 to 480 times over the course of her lifetime, most women know surprisingly little about their cycles. For women who take oral contraceptives, the menstrual cycle takes on an entirely different dimension: they don't need to count days (they only need to glance at their dispenser to see how many days are left in any given cycle). With the recent popularity of long-term contraceptives, some health experts are questioning whether women even need to bleed every month. Why not quarterly? Or once a year? What about, never? It's no wonder that the menstrual cycle is a mystery to so many.

What Happens Every Month

Every month, your body prepares for a potential pregnancy by developing an egg inside your ovaries. The egg is released and travels through the fallopian tube on its way to the uterus. If the egg isn't fertilized, the body sheds the uterine lining, causing a period that lasts an average of four to eight days. Then the body begins again—the uterine lining grows, an egg matures, is released, and so forth—for a cycle that lasts about twenty-eight days. If you get pregnant, the cycles cease. Once you're no longer pregnant, they start again. In between, about one or two weeks before your period, you get awful headaches, backaches, and a variety of other PMS symptoms.

Things go on this way until you get older and start perimenopause, the transitional period before menopause. At this point, your periods become more erratic, and you start to experience some menopause-like symptoms, such as hot flashes. After twelve months without periods, you are officially in menopause. But there is so much more to the menstrual cycle. For one thing, a period involves a complex interaction of hormone levels that rise and fall over the course of a cycle. These hormones not only control the biology of the menstrual cycle, but they impact how a woman feels: too much of one hormone may cause depression, while too much of another may cause anxiety. Monthly hormonal surges explain some of the emotional and psychological symptoms of PMS. In addition, there are a lot of variables, such as pregnancy, irregular ovulation, and contraceptives, that disrupt the typical menstrual cycle. There are also plenty of myths about menstruation that are just plain wrong, including the "fact" that every woman gets her period every twenty-eight days.

 Fact

Perimenopause is the stage that precedes menopause when the production of hormones such as estrogen and progesterone diminishes and becomes more irregular.

Menstrual Myths

In the United States, the average age of menarche, or the onset of menstruation, is twelve, while menopause typically occurs around fifty (the average age is 51.4). Sometime in the decade before menopause, nine out of ten women also experience perimenopause symptoms, in which their cycles become more erratic. That means a woman will have her period for nearly forty years—potentially, a very long time to suffer from PMS!

The complexity of the menstrual cycle and the fact that many women aren't terribly familiar with their bodies or their cycles help perpetuate a number of myths about a woman's period, including the following:

- Every woman's cycle is or should be twenty-eight days long.
- Every woman will or should ovulate every cycle.
- If a woman bleeds, she is not pregnant.
- A woman cannot ovulate or get pregnant when she has her period.
- The menstrual cycle starts when periods end.

The Truth

It's perfectly normal to have a cycle that lasts twenty-one, twenty-eight, or thirty-six days. Variation is normal, not only from woman to woman but also from month to month for any given woman. So you can have a cycle that is twenty-nine days one month and thirty-three days the next. The length of a menstrual cycle is tied to ovulation, which consistently occurs fourteen to sixteen days before a woman gets her period. This second half of the cycle is usually the same length. It is the first half, from the first day of your period until you ovulate, that can change from month to month.

Extreme variation, however, may signal an underlying health problem. If the pattern of your cycle goes wildly up and down—one month, twenty-one days, the next forty-five days, then eleven days, it can be a sign that you're not ovulating regularly. Similarly, if you get periods only two or three times a year, there could be a serious health issue involved. Note that variations in menstrual-cycle length are more common in young girls after they first get their periods and in older women who are undergoing perimenopause.

It's not unusual to skip a period once or twice a year. In fact, it's extremely common. This may be caused by stress, or, believe it or not, there may be no obvious reason. If you skip a period, it generally means you have not ovulated. What usually happens is that you ovulate next month and have a heavier flow than normal.

While technically not a period, some vaginal bleeding may occur while a woman is pregnant. A woman who takes contraceptives also does not get an actual period, but rather she experiences what's known as withdrawal bleeding.

Finally, if you've ever been confused when asked by your gynecologist when your last cycle began, here's the answer. Your period actually starts on the first day of bleeding, not on the day your period ends.

 # Fact

Many women have cycles when they don't ovulate and may not bleed. These are known as anovulatory cycles. Anovulatory cycles are not uncommon in the first twelve years after a girl starts to menstruate, in the first nine months after discontinuing oral contraceptives, during perimenopause, or in women who diet or exercise excessively.

Know Your Period: Biology Basics

The organs involved in menstruation are—surprise!—the brain (specifically, the hypothalamus), the pituitary gland, the ovaries, and the uterus.

- **Hypothalamus:** This region of the brain regulates the menstrual cycle (it also regulates thirst, hunger, sleep patterns, libido, and other endocrine functions) by releasing a chemical messenger called follicle-stimulating hormone-releasing factor (FSH-RF) to stimulate the pituitary gland.
- **Pituitary gland:** This "master gland" releases the follicle-stimulating hormone (FSH), plus a little luteinizing hormone (LH), into the bloodstream, which cause egg-containing follicles in the ovaries to mature.
- **Ovaries:** These two small glands, roughly the size and shape of almonds, store a woman's eggs, each in its own sac called a follicle. Under the influence of FSH and LH, the ovaries grow and mature ten to twenty follicles, until one is fully mature (the others simply die away) and bursts, causing ovulation.

- **Uterus:** This pear-shaped organ grows a lining, called the endometrium, which nourishes a fertilized egg during pregnancy. If an egg is not fertilized, the lining sloughs away, causing a period.

The Hormone Connection

At their very core, menstruation and, by extension, PMS are hormonal events, controlled by the fluctuation of hormones in a woman's body. Four hormones work together to control a menstrual cycle:

1. Follicle-stimulating hormone (secreted by the pituitary gland)
2. Luteinizing hormone (secreted by the pituitary gland)
3. Estrogen (secreted by the ovaries)
4. Progesterone (secreted by the ovaries)

The levels of these hormones rise and fall during the month, and depending on their levels, they can trigger PMS symptoms. Chapters 5 through 8 discuss the most common PMS symptoms.

The Cycle Starts

At the start of the period, on Day One, when bleeding begins, FSH and LH are at their lowest levels of the entire cycle, which also cause low levels of progesterone and estrogen. This first half of the cycle is known as the follicular, proliferative, or estrogenic phase because this is when estrogen, secreted by the ovaries, begins to rise and triggers the growth of the uterine lining.

Mid-Cycle

Mid-cycle, as ovulation approaches, hormone levels continue to increase: LH and FSH levels rise, as does the level of estrogen. When the follicle starts to mature, the ovaries secrete a surge of progesterone in addition to the estrogen. This triggers ovulation, and this is when LH, FSH, and estrogen are at their highest levels. Depending on the length of a woman's cycle, ovulation can occur on Day Seven (in a twenty-one-day cycle), Day Fourteen (in a twenty-eight-day cycle), Day Twenty-one (in a thirty-five-day cycle), or somewhere in between.

Ovulation and the Luteal Phase

Once ovulation occurs, the luteal phase of the cycle begins. It lasts about fourteen days. Immediately, FSH returns to its base level while estrogen and LH begin to fall more gradually. In contrast, progesterone increases. Progesterone is secreted by the released follicle, now known as the corpus luteum, so that the lining in the uterus will produce fluids that nourish the egg. If a woman becomes pregnant, the levels of estrogen and progesterone stay elevated to maintain the pregnancy, but if no pregnancy occurs, progesterone falls and causes the endometrial lining to shed. Thus the period begins. In essence, the levels of estrogen and progesterone rise at different rates during a woman's menstrual cycle to optimize pregnancy and implantation.

The Chain of Events

The cascade of events between the organs and hormones involved in menstruation goes something like this:

1. Hypothalamus releases FSH-RF to stimulate the pituitary gland.
2. The pituitary gland releases FSH.
3. The ovaries begin to grow follicles, which release two hormones, estrogen and progesterone, into the woman's bloodstream. When the follicle matures, the ovaries release a surge of progesterone.
4. The estrogen and progesterone stimulate the hypothalamus to send out two chemical messengers: FSH-RF and luteinizing hormone–releasing factor (LH-RF).
5. In response, the pituitary gland sends out FHS and LH simultaneously.

6. The surge of LH causes the most mature follicle to burst open and release an egg. This is called ovulation.

7. The follicle, now called the corpus luteum, secretes estrogen in decreasing amounts and progesterone in increasing amounts.

8. Under the influence of progesterone, the uterine lining secretes a fluid that nourishes the egg.

9. If pregnancy occurs, the egg attaches itself to the uterine wall. The corpus luteum continues to release progesterone and estrogen, and the body produces a hormone called HCG (which is what early pregnancy tests detect in a woman's urine).

10. If the egg is not fertilized, the corpus luteum degenerates. The falling levels of progesterone cause the spiral arteries of the endometrial lining to close off, stopping blood flow to the surface of the lining. The blood pools in the lining and eventually bursts it. This blood, along with the endometrial lining, forms the menstrual flow.

11. FSH, LH, estrogen, and progesterone drop to base levels.

12. When estrogen falls below a certain level, the hypothalamus once again stimulates the pituitary gland with FSH-RF.

The Ovulation Connection

Ovulation is the key moment in a woman's cycle: the follicle is mature, and the body is flush with hormones. At this point, PMS symptoms usually appear, particularly around the time that progesterone drops sharply. Progesterone affects the body in several ways, including helping maintain feelings of well-being, relaxing muscles, and helping the body transform food into energy. So when progesterone levels drop one or two weeks before the period starts, headaches, crabbiness, and bloating kick in.

Progesterone, which can be considered the female equivalent of testosterone, has a great many functions in the body, including:

- Regulating the thyroid gland
- Raising the body's core temperature
- Acting as an anti-inflammatory and regulating immune response
- Acting as an antidepressant
- Helping the body use fat for energy
- Affecting the body's sodium-to-water balance
- Reducing spasm and relaxing smooth muscle
- Normalizing blood sugar levels
- Increasing fertility
- Helping the body absorb vitamins and minerals
- Enhancing the libido
- Promoting bone building

The Highs (and Lows) of Estrogen

It is probably more accurate to say that low levels of progesterone, combined with elevated levels of estrogen, appear to cause many PMS symptoms. The body functions well when estrogen and progesterone are in proper balance, but when that balance is compromised, as it can be during the luteal phase (the second half) of a typical menstrual cycle, a woman will experience side effects of the imbalance.

Studies have shown that if estrogen exceeds a normal estrogen/progesterone ratio, PMS symptoms increase. For example, estrogen interferes with the body's thyroid function, while progesterone enhances it.

Cells in the body depend on hormones secreted by the thyroid gland to regulate their metabolism, and poor thyroid function decreases the body's ability to use carbohydrates, fats, and proteins. So, high estrogen levels inhibit thyroid hormone levels, which, in turn, cause cravings and increased appetite because the body is not effectively using food. Low thyroid levels can also cause depression, weakness, and fatigue.

Fact

> The thyroid, one of the larger endocrine glands in the body, regulates the body's metabolism (or how fast it burns energy). The thyroid is connected to reproductive function, and that connection may be tighter in women than in men. Women may be more vulnerable to thyroid impairment, predisposing them to rapid mood cycles.

Similarly, research has shown that estrogen intensifies the effect of aldosterone, a hormone that helps regulate levels of sodium and potassium in the body. In contrast, progesterone blocks the effects of aldosterone, so high estrogen levels, combined with low progesterone levels, lead to fluid retention or bloating.

Too much estrogen in the body also decreases endorphin levels in the brain, causing depression and anxiety. Endorphins are the feel-good chemicals in the brain that regulate or elevate mood. Studies have shown that women with PMS commonly have low endorphin levels.

Cramps and PMS

Though it may be surprising, cramps are not typically associated with PMS. Painful periods, known as dysmenorrhea, are quite common; they are caused by uterine contractions, which is how the body expels the endometrial lining. In other words, the uterus contracts in order to shed the endometrial lining and thus causes cramps.

In contrast, premenstrual syndrome is related to hormone fluctuations and may be aggravated by vitamin and mineral deficiencies, depressive disorders, stress, and multiple psychological disturbances. A woman can have primary dysmenorrhea, which means there is no underlying cause for the pain, or secondary dysmenorrhea, in which pain is caused by another medical condition such as endometriosis or fibroids.

Many women experience cramping during their periods without the bloating, depression, anxiety, or headaches that are more common to PMS. Some women are more disposed to cramping simply because their uterus contracts more than the next woman's. Cramps may also be related to low levels of calcium. Experts believe that prostaglandins, which are hormone-like substances involved in pain and inflammation, may trigger menstrual cramps. (Chapters 5, 6, 7, 9, and 18 also discuss prostaglandins.) Women with PMS may or may not experience cramps.

When Does PMS Occur?

As noted previously, PMS symptoms appear in the second half of a woman's menstrual cycle, most likely because of the sharp drop in progesterone levels. But, as with the length of a normal menstrual cycle, variation is normal.

Essential

Hormones and chemical transmitters in the brain, called neurotransmitters, perform interrelated functions in PMS. The hormones estrogen and progesterone regulate the menstrual cycle, and the neurotransmitters serotonin and gamma-aminobutyric acid (GABA) protect against PMS symptoms.

In the usual scenario, PMS symptoms appear seven to ten days before menstruation and get progressively worse until the day the woman gets her period, at which point they either cease immediately or taper off more gradually (usually within four days of getting a period). A small number of women, between 5 and 10 percent, experience a short burst of PMS symptoms around ovulation. PMS experts believe this may be related to the fall in estrogen that occurs around the middle of a woman's menstrual cycle.

 ## Fact

Estrogen is a hormone compound. Three hormones make up estrogen: estradiol, estriol, and estrone. Estradiol predominates in women during their reproductive years, while postmenopausal women have more estrone in their bodies.

Some women complain of symptoms that begin shortly after ovulation and continue throughout their periods. Given that ovulation can occur two weeks before a woman's period and a period can last eight days, this means three full weeks of PMS! In some women, experts say, this near-constant experience of PMS gets progressively worse and can appear to be a mood disorder.

In another interesting twist, PMS also appears to occur frequently and more severely in women who are thirty or older. Many women complain that their symptoms get progressively worse with age. However, given that PMS can strike a menstruating woman of any age—usually starting anywhere from about two years after a girl starts menstruating, or about age fourteen, all the way through to menopause—this increase in severity has some experts puzzled. One theory is that women forty and older are really experiencing some of the symptoms of menopause or perimenopause but confuse them with PMS. Another is that older women see health-care providers for non-pregnancy-related reasons more frequently and therefore have more opportunities to seek help for PMS. Finally, a third theory is that the emotional and mood swings so common with PMS are written off in teenagers as part of adolescence. The truth of the matter is that there's not enough information about PMS to tell for certain why older women are more likely to have more severe PMS.

Essential

> The mid-cycle drop in estradiol is thought to cause PMS symptoms around ovulation in some women.

What It Means for You

Getting a handle on your menstrual cycle—understanding it and being familiar with the changes you experience from month to month—is the first step you can take to manage PMS symptoms. One concrete way to do this is to keep a menstrual diary. Many women who want to get pregnant, especially those who suspect they may have fertility problems, use menstrual diaries to track ovulation and to time intercourse so they get pregnant. The concept here is the same, even if the intent is simply to know the length of your cycles, the length of your luteal phase, and whether you ovulate regularly.

Use that same approach to track your PMS symptoms. Jot down the symptoms you experience and when they occur. Note the major stressors in your life: Are there issues at home or at work that may be aggravating your symptoms? How long have you experienced symptoms? Recently? For a few months? For the last several years? Prepare yourself for questions your doctor might ask you about your cycle and your symptoms.

Fact

> It can take a long time to diagnose PMS! One study showed that women sought help for over an average 5.33 years (and saw an average of 3.75 doctors) for their symptoms before being diagnosed with PMS.

Not only is the process of tracking your symptoms and circumstances a great way to build awareness, it's a necessary step in the medical diagnosis process. Doctors prefer to see hard evidence of symptoms before providing a diagnosis. (Chapter 13 outlines how to keep a PMS diary and a menstrual diary and provides samples for easy reference.)

Going Forward

Once you know your menstrual cycle and recognize your symptoms, you can move on to treatment. The first tactic is usually to self-treat PMS. Perhaps changing your diet, taking up exercise, or adding dietary supplements such as magnesium or calcium will relieve the worst of your symptoms. If self-treatment doesn't do the trick, that's when you should see a physician, counselor, psychologist, or psychiatrist.

Remember, studies show that only 31 percent of all the women who believe they have PMS get a positive diagnosis from their doctor. The remaining 69 percent may have PMDD or other health or psychological issues, be undergoing menopause, or have symptoms that are brought on by stress or lifestyle.

When PMS affects your life, it is up to you to take charge and get help. While there has been significant progress in recent years, most notably with the official recognition of PMDD as a mood disorder, there is still some reluctance on the part of medical experts to recognize and diagnose PMS in some women. The understanding of the condition is simply too murky and other possible culprits are too numerous.

CHAPTER 3

Is Biology Going
to Get You?

PMS SYMPTOMS DO HAVE physiologic causes, but they're also caused by psychological factors and stress. Over the last twenty years or so, as experts have gotten a better understanding of PMS, the debate about PMS has become more productive. Instead of questioning whether symptoms are real, as was common in the 1970s and 1980s, experts now debate the disorder's specific causes. Which hormones, health issues, or mood disorders cause or contribute to PMS? Some of these questions can be answered by understanding your biological likelihood—if any—of getting PMS.

Who Gets PMS?

The short answer is women who are menstruating (and ovulating), from about age fourteen (or about two years after the average onset of menstruation) through their early fifties, until they undergo perimenopause and menopause. Although a woman of any age can have PMS, it often first appears when a woman is in her mid-twenties, and many women report their symptoms get progressively worse as they get older. PMS symptoms may also be exacerbated in women who are stressed, have more children, suffer from mood disorders, or have relatives with PMS.

Depression, a risk factor for PMS, also is most likely to appear in women in their late twenties to mid-thirties, so there may be a confluence of age, depression, and PMS as women age. In other words, women in this age bracket are more likely to become depressed and also to get PMS; however, a casual relationship has yet to be demonstrated.

 # Question

> **Why do PMS symptoms first appear in young adult women?**
> Although it can affect women of any age, PMS often first strikes women when they are young adults in their mid-twenties. PMS tends to occur in women with more years of regular cycles, and while teen-agers can get PMS, they may be less likely to do so because teenagers have more irregular cycles (and are not ovulating regularly).

Stress

Stress, so common in our culture today, also appears to be a big culprit in whether a woman gets PMS, and how severe it is. A 1990 British study by Warner P. Bancroft found that after six years of natural cycles, women with high stress levels were more likely to report symptoms of PMS. Other studies have found that women who report PMS also indicate they experience high stress from work, financial strain, dissatisfaction with marriage, busy schedules, and family conflict. Is this because stress makes women perceive their symptoms more acutely? Or are stress and PMS biologically connected? Some research does indicate a biological connection. (Chapter 10 discusses stress as a risk factor for PMS in more detail.)

Culture

Believe it or not, your culture influences how you perceive PMS symptoms, including which symptoms you believe are worst and how severe you believe them to be. Women who live in the United States or in Western Europe perceive PMS differently than women who live in China, for example.

A number of researchers from different disciples, including law, have argued that PMS is a culture-specific syndrome limited to

Western countries. In 2002, Joan Christler, a professor of psychology at Connecticut College, detailed some of the culture-specific thinking about PMS. She notes, for example, that much of the research has been conducted by scientists in a few Western countries, including Australia, given its European heritage, Canada, Germany, the Netherlands, Britain, Sweden, and the United States. Surveys by the World Health Organization also indicate that women in Western Europe, Australia, and North America are the most likely to report menstrual cycle–related complaints (except cramps). In contrast, women in Asia are not only less likely to report their symptoms as severe, but when they do report PMS symptoms, their symptoms differ from those reported by women in Western countries.

 Fact

A culture-bound or culture-specific syndrome is a combination of symptoms, both psychiatric and physical, that is a recognizable disease or dysfunction only within a specific society or culture.

While studies detailed that women all over the world experience similar symptoms related to their menstrual cycle, they reveal that not all women perceive the symptoms in the same way and that what some women consider as PMS, others do not. For example, studies have found that Asian women report pain as the most significant symptom in PMS, while Western women say it's depression. In addition, women in Hong Kong and Mainland China report increased sensitivity to cold as a PMS symptom, while American women do not. In a 2002 study of American health maintenance organizations, women of Asian descent reported fewer PMS symptoms than Caucasian women, while Hispanic-American women reported more severe symptoms. Experts like Christler believe that cultural perspective influences how a woman sees her symptoms and whether she sees them as just part of being female or as part of a medical disorder that can (or should) be treated. "Only in Western societies (and more often in some than in others) do women think their premenstrual emotional state is abnormal and might signify a need for professional intervention," Christler writes in a 2002 article in the journal *Annual Review of Sex Research*.

Essential

Earlier studies, from the 1970s, reported a difference between a woman's religion and whether she complained of PMS. In 1973, Karen E. Paige, a psychologist at the University of California, Davis, surveyed women and found that strict Catholics and Orthodox Jews had the most severe menstrual complaints. These religions also strongly supported traditional feminine role models.

Is It Biological Destiny?

In the last twenty or thirty years, researchers have moved from looking at PMS as a cultural issue to examining it increasingly from a biological perspective.

Although researchers have not yet established a definite genetic link for PMS, there does appear to be a genetic link to sensitivity to hormonal changes. Studies show, for example, that identical twins are twice as likely to have PMS than fraternal twins. So while no PMS gene has been found, experts agree that, biologically speaking, some women are more likely to get PMS than others.

Some women appear to be more sensitive to hormonal fluctuations and are more likely to experience PMS. A recent National Institute of Mental Health study showed that women with a preexisting vulnerability to PMS experienced relief from symptoms when their sex hormones were suppressed, but once the hormones were reintroduced, they again developed symptoms. In contrast, women without a history of PMS reported no effects from hormonal manipulation.

Fact

In 1977, British endocrinologist Katharina Dalton observed that women who lived alone were much less likely to suffer from PMS than women who lived with men.

The prevailing theory among experts is that women with low levels of the brain chemical serotonin are particularly sensitive to changes in the level of progesterone, which might lead to symptoms of PMS. Experts also believe that some women may have a genetic predisposition to get PMDD. The neurotransmitter serotonin affects emotions, behavior, and thought, and is known to play a role in depression. It also appears to play a role in PMDD. A 2001 Canadian study, published in the *Archives of Women's Health*, is one of several studies that suggest women with PMDD may have a dysfunction of the serotonin transporter gene. However, the evidence for this theory is not conclusive. A more recent study, published in November 2006 in the *American Journal of Obstetrics & Gynecology*, compared fifty-three women diagnosed with PMDD with fifty-two healthy women and found no evidence that the genes that control serotonin are associated with PMDD. The conclusion is that some women may have a biological tendency to get PMDD, but experts haven't conclusively determined why.

Researchers are looking at the following possible culprits of PMS and PMDD:

- **Serotonin:** A chemical in the nervous system believed to play an important role in the regulation of mood, sleep sexuality, and appetite, as well as in disorders such as migraines, anxiety, and depression. Low levels of serotonin or a dysfunction in the serotonin transporter gene are thought to be responsible for PMS and PMDD.

- **Gamma-aminobutyric acid (GABA):** The body's main chemical messenger is found in the nervous system. There is increasing evidence it plays a role in mood disorders.

Experts once believed that PMS and PMDD were caused by a hormonal imbalance in women. Now, the prevailing belief is that normal cyclical changes in the sex hormones trigger the conditions. The cyclical changes dramatically shift the levels of progesterone and estrogen, essentially putting women's bodies into a tailspin. Those with great sensitivity to the fluctuations experience severe PMS or PMDD. In other words, normal hormonal changes trigger PMS and PMDD.

Question

What is genetic vulnerability?
Genetic vulnerability is an inherited risk (or risks) for an individual to develop a specific illness. Genetic vulnerability does not mean an individual will get the illness or condition, only that he or she has genetic risk factors for it. Women with a genetic vulnerability to PMS have an inherited sensitivity to hormonal changes that may lead to PMS symptoms.

Key Risk Factors

Aside from having regular menstrual cycles, there are a number of other well-known risk factors that predispose a woman to experience PMS:

- Depression
- A personality or mood disorder
- Family history
- High salt intake
- A diet high in sugar

- Vitamin B6 deficiency
- Magnesium deficiency
- Calcium deficiency
- High caffeine consumption
- Lack of exercise

Some of these risk factors, such as depression, mood disorders, or family history, are outside a woman's control, while others, like diet and exercise, are within her power to change and improve. It's important to know which risk factors may apply to you to treat PMS appropriately. For example, if your diet is healthful and you exercise regularly and in the appropriate amounts, you may look to medical or psychological treatment more quickly than those women who need to become more physically active and to adjust their diet. Conversely, realizing that diet may be the cause of your symptoms can empower you to take control of your PMS instead of becoming resigned to a condition that's treatable only by a doctor or a counselor.

Less well-known factors associated with PMS include:

- Having more children versus having fewer children
- Seasonal affective disorder, also known as SAD
- Tubal ligation surgery (i.e., having the fallopian tubes tied)

Several studies have shown a correlation between alcoholism and PMS. Evidence suggests that some women, especially those with a family history of alcohol abuse, tend to drink more before their periods. Seasonal affective disorder has also been shown to have a correlation with PMS. Interestingly, alcoholism and SAD, like PMS, seem to be manifestations of an individual's low serotonin levels, sometimes called serotonin deficiency syndrome.

Tubal ligation surgery, a surgical procedure in which a woman's fallopian tubes are tied off or obstructed, is also associated with PMS. Some women find that they experience severe PMS symptoms after having their tubes tied, even if they did not have PMS symptoms prior to surgery or only suffered mild PMS. This is known as post tubal ligation syndrome (the diagnosis of which has been surrounded by controversy). Its symptoms include irregular, heavy periods, a loss of libido, and severe PMS symptoms. However, the association between PMS and tubal ligation surgery remains controversial. A 1991 study published in the *Journal of Reproductive Medicine* by researchers at the State University of New York, Buffalo, failed to show a link between PMS and tubal ligation. Nevertheless, many women continue to report increased severity in PMS symptoms after tubal ligation surgery despite a lack of medical evidence to support their claims.

Question

What is serotonin deficiency syndrome?
Although this is a popular term, especially in alternative medicine, many experts dispute the notion of a serotonin deficiency syndrome. Dr. Thomas M. Kramer has argued that there is no such thing as a deficit or surplus of serotonin in the body. Rather, neurotransmitters such as serotonin exist in the brain in relatively constant amounts, and patients have brain cells with an impaired ability to accept serotonin on either side of their membrane.

Children

Can the stress of raising children make your PMS symptoms more severe? Some research may support that possibility. A 1988 study of sixty women by E. W. Freeman and colleagues at the University of Pennsylvania found that women with more children have more severe PMS symptoms. The researchers believe that family and daily stress factors play a big role in PMS.

A 2004 study of ninety-six women showed that the more children a woman had, the more likely she was to complain of PMS. Eighty percent of women with one or two children reported PMS-related behavior changes, but all—100 percent—of the women with more than two children reported behavioral changes, such as depression and agitation. In contrast, only one-third of women without children were affected.

Work and Education

A multiyear study by the World Health Organization, conducted between 1973 and 1982, found that perceptions and patterns of menstruation were not influenced by a woman's geographic location but by other factors, such as socioeconomic status and education, that played a part in how symptoms were perceived.

A 1985 study found that homemakers and women with lower levels of education reported more PMS symptoms than women who worked outside the home or those with higher levels of education. These findings were supported by a 2004 study of ninety-six women.

Stress and other lesser-known factors may be worth considering if you're trying to discover why you suffer from PMS and are still stumped after considering the usual suspects.

Family History

Did your mother have PMS? Does your sister? Perhaps your cousins or your aunts? Are you worried your daughter will have it someday? Or maybe she suffers from it already and you worry that you're to blame? A family history provides clues about how—or if—a disorder will manifest itself in an individual. A history of PMS in your family strongly suggests that you will also have PMS.

Researchers aren't exactly sure why PMS runs in families, but they theorize it has to do with having inherited a greater-than-normal sensitivity to hormonal fluctuations. But there are a couple of other interesting points to consider. For one, the connection between PMS, depression, mood, anxiety and bipolar disorders, and family history is intriguing. Not only is family history a big risk factor for PMS, it's also a significant risk factor for mood disorders and anxiety. So if your mother had a history of depression, she also had a greater-than-average chance of having PMS. The same goes for you: not only are you more likely to become depressed, you're also more likely to have PMS—for both conditions, family history is a major risk factor. Experts estimate that as many as 50 percent of women with PMS will be found to have an underlying mood disorder. Because the connection between depression and PMS is fairly strong, if you have depression, you're predisposed to getting PMS, regardless of whether someone in your family had it as well.

Inheriting Stress, Inheriting PMS?

Stress, like depression, has a correlation with both PMS and family history. Genes play a big part in how a person reacts to stress; recent research suggests that babies can even "inherit" stress while in the womb. A study on pregnant women and stress showed that high levels of the stress hormone cortisol may cross the placenta and affect the fetus. High stress levels worsen PMS symptoms and can even cause periods to stop. So if your family history includes a high sensitivity to stress, you are also more susceptible to high stress—and its negative effects on PMS. One of the best strategies to reduce stress is regular exercise. (Chapter 15 discusses exercise as a self-treatment for PMS.)

Essential

Stress causes the brain to release hormones that trigger a fight-or-flight response, heart and blood pressure to rise, and breathing to quicken. Once the stress-inducing crisis passes, hormone levels drop and the body returns to normal. In people who are vulnerable to stress, such as those with depression, however, the hormone levels do not quite return to normal. Over time, this kind of low-level, chronic stress affects the organs.

Nurture Versus Nature

Other theories on family history and PMS focus on upbringing rather than genetics. These theories hold that women who suffer from PMS did not learn to eat correctly or to exercise properly while growing up. Instead, their family legacy includes a diet high in salt, sugar, and caffeine and low in vitamins and minerals and an aversion to exercise, all of which exacerbate PMS symptoms.

Age: Older Isn't Necessarily Better

As you age, the more likely it is that you will experience PMS symptoms, report them to your doctor, and seek treatment for them. Being in your thirties or older is associated with a whole host of factors that influence whether you have PMS: a long, steady pattern of regular periods, a drop in hormone levels, and a critical time when the incidence of depression peaks.

Continuous Menstrual Cycles

Having a history of uninterrupted menstrual cycles—that is, a several-year span of not being pregnant and not using oral contraceptives—may predispose a woman to develop PMS. A 1990 study published in the *British Journal of Psychiatry* of nearly 5,500 readers of a U.K. women's magazine found that women who used oral contraceptives were less likely to report PMS than nonusers and that the longer a woman experienced continual menstrual cycles, the more likely she was to have PMS.

PMS symptoms that begin when a woman is in her late thirties or early forties may be linked to a reduction in androgens, or male hormones. A woman in her forties only produces about half the level of androgens that a woman in her twenties produces.

 Fact

Androgen is the hormone compound responsible for male characteristics, such as large muscles, a deep voice, and obvious or excessive facial hair. All women produce androgen (just as all men produce estrogen) but in much smaller amounts than men.

Two principal androgens are testosterone and DHT. In women, testosterone is produced by the ovaries and the adrenal glands (which sit atop the kidneys). Testosterone is considered the precursor to estrogen; women produce increased amounts of testosterone in puberty. As they age, women produce decreasing amounts.

Mood Disorders

Having a mood disorder is one of the greatest risk factors for developing PMS and PMDD (which is itself characterized as a mood disorder). Women are nearly twice as likely as men to develop a mood disorder. Researchers believe that genetic, biological, hormonal, psychological, social, and interpersonal factors play a role in why women are more likely to become depressed. The fluctuations of a woman's reproductive hormones impact mood, and mood disorders tend to present differently across genders. For example, women are more likely to suffer from depression, while men are more likely to experience mania.

 Question

What is a mood disorder?
A mood disorder involves patterns of perception, behavior, and relating that are inflexible and socially inappropriate. Mood disorders typically include major depressive disorder (MDD) and bipolar disorder.

PMS and PMDD expert Jean Endicott, Ph.D., of New York's Columbia University, believes that during the premenstrual phase of her cycle, a woman is more vulnerable to severe depression or the worsening of an ongoing period of depression.

The main mood disorders include:

- Major depressive disorder
- Bipolar disorder

- Seasonal affective disorder
- Schizoaffective disorder

Depression

Clinical depression, also known as major depression, is a state of sadness and despair so acute it disrupts an individual's ability to participate in daily activities and function socially. More than just a feeling of being depressed, clinical depression is a medical diagnosis. Someone who is clinically depressed must either have a loss of interest or pleasure in all daily activities or be in a depressed mood for at least two weeks. Depression is strongly associated with PMS. (Chapter 8 covers depression and its role in PMS in more detail.)

Symptoms of clinical depression include (but are not limited to):

- Change in appetite
- Fatigue
- Marked weight gain or loss
- Feelings of overwhelming sadness, fear, or emptiness
- Anxiety
- Trouble concentrating

As noted earlier, the association between depression and PMS is very strong. Depression first hits many women when they're in their thirties. This is also the time when many women first experience PMS symptoms.

 Fact

Dysthymic disorder, also called dysthymia, is a depression characterized by a lack of enjoyment or pleasure in life that continues for at least two years. It is less severe than clinical depression but typically lasts much longer.

Bipolar Disorders

Unlike depression with its constant and overwhelming feelings of helplessness and anxiety, bipolar disorders feature alternating episodes of mania and depression. Bipolar disorder is caused by changes in a person's brain chemistry. Women who have bipolar disorder are more likely to have PMS.

During a manic state, the person will have a severely elevated mood—high energy, talkative, and hyperactive but frequently grandiose, irritable, and belligerent. Many times, individuals with bipolar disorder will experience rapid cycling, or quick shifts, between the two extreme states, anywhere from having four episodes per year to moods that cycle daily or even hourly.

Not surprisingly, there is a spectrum of bipolar disorders; some patients have the most severe symptoms, including hallucinations and delusions, while others experience hypomania, a more mild form of mania in which the individual experiences mostly feelings of euphoria. Some bipolar disorders may include mixed states (some manic symptoms along with some depressive symptoms).

Symptoms of bipolar disorder include:

- Elevated mood
- Irritability
- Racing thoughts
- Grandiose thinking
- Religiosity
- Disrupted sleep patterns
- Obsessional traits

Seasonal Affective Disorder

Seasonal affective disorder, or SAD, is a type of depression brought on by a deficiency of sunlight. Having SAD is a risk factor for PMS. As the name suggests, SAD is seasonal, occurring during fall and winter. The disorder affects up to 10 million people each year—75 to 80 percent of whom are women thirty and older. Some symptoms of PMS are similar to those of SAD, including depression, fatigue, trouble concentrating, and an increased appetite, especially for carbohydrates.

So what, exactly, is the connection between a lack of sunshine and depression and PMS? In one word: serotonin. Sunlight helps the body produce serotonin, and during the shorter, cloudier days of fall and winter, serotonin levels fall, while levels of the sleep hormone melatonin rise. As a result, those with SAD feel depressed, tired, and sleepy. Women with SAD can also feel more intense PMS or PMDD symptoms.

 ## Fact

Melatonin regulates the body's sleep cycle and has a calming effect. At night and during winter, melatonin levels naturally increase.

SAD is a risk factor for women with PMS: women with SAD are more likely to develop PMS, and women with PMS are more likely to suffer from SAD. One study found a high prevalence of PMDD in women who suffered from SAD.

Postpartum Depression

Postpartum depression affects between 10 and 15 percent of new mothers. It's caused by the rapid and severe hormonal changes that take place just after childbirth. Postpartum depression, or PPD, is a severe form of the "baby blues" that commonly affects many new moms. It can occur anytime in the first six months after childbirth. If untreated, PPD may last up to a year.

There is research that shows a link between the PMS and PPD. In fact, one of the risk factors for PPD is having severe PMS. According to the American Psychiatric Association, typical PPD symptoms include a loss of interest in life, less motivation to do things, a loss of appetite, feeling restless, irritable, or anxious, and in severe cases, being afraid of harming yourself or the baby.

Schizoaffective Disorder

This psychiatric illness combines the symptoms of schizophrenia and the symptoms of a mood disorder. As with other mood disorders, it is a risk factor for PMS. Psychotic symptoms include delusions, hallucinations, and disorganized speech (for example, incoherence), while affective symptoms include depression or mania. A person with schizoaffective disorder suffers from depression or bipolar disorder but also experiences psychotic symptoms without prominent mood symptoms for at least two weeks. More women than men are diagnosed with schizoaffective disorder, and the illness tends to begin between the ages of sixteen and thirty.

Researchers are relatively certain that schizoaffective disorder involves a chemical imbalance of neurotransmitters, and stress seems to serve as a trigger, but they're not sure what causes this disorder. Some argue that schizoaffective disorder is linked to schizophrenia, while others link it to mood disorders. However, both genetic and environmental factors are thought to be involved.

Why You Shouldn't Worry

Having PMS does not mean you have a mood disorder. While mood disorders are a PMS risk factor, only a very small number of women are affected. Remember, only 3 to 8 percent of all women with PMS symptoms have PMDD, which is considered a mood disorder, and fewer than half of a percent of this small number have a different mood disorder, such as depression, that is misdiagnosed as PMDD. So if you're feeling irritable and upset, it's far more likely that you have PMS than a serious mental illness like depression or an anxiety disorder.

CHAPTER 4

Types of PMS:
An Alphabet of Choices

THE MISCONCEPTION IN WESTERN culture—and indeed, among many women—is that PMS is uniform and that everyone who has PMS feels the same way. The reality is that PMS symptoms are so varied that the syndrome can look very different from woman to woman. However, some symptoms, such as bloating or mood swings, are more common than others, and many women have constellations of certain symptoms. Some PMS experts have identified patterns of symptoms that appear together. They have also tried to account for why some women are more prone to one set of symptoms than another.

There's Not Just One Kind of PMS

A cursory search on the Internet will bring up a list of different types of PMS: anxiety, depression, bloating, cravings, and headaches. Each of these types has several associated symptoms and, of course, several remedies to relieve those symptoms. However, it's important to understand that dividing PMS into specific types is a popular, rather than a medical, practice. Many health-care practitioners and experts who discuss PMS types advocate alternative medicine rather than conventional Western medicine.

Is it PMS?

You may be convinced that your breast pain, mood swings, and bloating are caused by your oncoming period, but you may be wrong.

There are a number of conditions with symptoms that resemble or mimic those of PMS, such as an unrecognized pelvic inflammation or thyroid disorders. These conditions are unrelated to PMS but are often confused with it, and women seeking treatment for PMS feel stymied when their symptoms don't seem to be relieved. These conditions include:

- Fibrocystic breast condition (which is also subject to premenstrual magnification)
- Endometriosis, which can cause lower abdominal pain
- Unrecognized pelvic inflammation
- Dysmenorrhea (cramps that can also cause nausea and diarrhea)
- Diabetes (which causes excessive thirst and hunger)
- Endocrine disorders such as an overactive thyroid
- Mood disorders

However, grouping PMS symptoms into clusters can be useful: it allows women to better understand their own experience, helps narrow treatment choices that address their specific symptoms, and may open alternatives to standard medicine, should they wish to try them.

Two Schools of Thought

There are two schools of thought on PMS types: conventional and alternative. The first does not divide PMS into types, while the second does.

Most conventional experts—generally, these include physicians, psychiatrists, and psychologists—prefer to speak about a range of PMS symptoms, as opposed to dividing PMS into distinct types. Conventional medicine does divide PMS symptoms into groups, which generally include physical, behavioral, and psychological symptoms. However, depending on the study author or the professional medical group, the names of the symptom groups, as well as the specific symptoms they include, can vary and may confuse the average person.

For example, a 1998 article in the journal *American Family Physician* defines four groups of PMS symptoms: affective, cognitive/performance, fluid retention, and general somatic.

 Fact

Somatic is a term that means "of or pertaining to the body." In general, the terms *somatic* or *physical* can be used to describe the same symptoms. Somatic/physical symptoms include dizziness, fatigue, nausea, and insomnia.

An article in 2003 by a different author in the same journal discusses only three groups of symptoms: behavioral, psychological, and physical. For the average woman, this inconsistency simply means she needs to be vigilant when it comes to learning about and understanding PMS to avoid confusing herself or her caregiver when describing her symptoms.

 Question

What are the differences between affective, cognitive, and psychological symptoms?
Affective symptoms impact mood, while cognitive symptoms impact reasoning, perception, and understanding. Psychological symptoms include both affective and cognitive components. So, for example, depression is considered both an affective symptom and a psychological symptom. In contrast, confusion or forgetfulness is a cognitive and psychological symptom.

As far as conventional medicine is concerned, grouping symptoms is not considered central to successful treatment and treating one set of symptoms often yields improvement in another set of symptoms. Unlike the four or five popular types of PMS that exist, the only official medical subtype of PMS is PMDD.

Who Defines Types?

Unlike conventional PMS experts, many nutritionists and practitioners or proponents of alternative medicine promote the notion that there are different kinds of PMS based on clusters of symptoms. They also tend to identify the culprits responsible for each type of PMS, such as an imbalance of hormones (a low ratio of progesterone compared with a high level of estrogen), mineral deficiencies, or poor diet.

⌐. Essential

In 1980, Guy Abraham, an obstetrician/gynecologist who founded Optimox, Inc., a nutritional supplement company in Torrance, California, divided PMS into four different types: Type A: Anxiety, Type C: Carbohydrate or Cravings, Type D: Depression, and Type H: Hyperhydration.

Indeed, the bulk of the literature about PMS types is from alternative medicine experts, as well as from nutritional supplement companies. These individuals and groups often promote natural remedies, such as herbs, to combat the specific group of symptoms in each type of PMS. Women interested in alternative therapies may find the information useful, but individuals interested in conventional medical treatment must be aware that the descriptions of PMS and its causes vary widely depending on the viewpoint and treatment philosophy of each "expert."

Opposing Views

Are these two views inherently contradictory? The evidence is unclear. One question centers around whether PMS symptoms in any given woman are consistent enough from month to month to be considered a "type" of PMS? To successfully treat a "type" of PMS, the practitioner would have to demonstrate that the symptoms appear month in and month out in a given woman. To date, there is research to support both sides of the story: that symptoms are stable and that they shift.

For example, a 1997 study of sixteen women found that over three cycles, the women's physical and mood symptoms showed remarkable stability from cycle to cycle. The study participants reported not only the same symptoms but ranked them similarly in terms of severity. Mood symptoms such as anxiety, irritability, and mood lability were the least likely to change from month to month and were also the most disabling.

 Question

What is mood lability?
Lability is the quality of shifting or changing rapidly. PMS researchers refer to mood lability to describe unstable or quickly changing moods.

According to this study's findings, a woman who feels anxiety, bloating, and fatigue in one month, with anxiety as the most severe symptom, is very likely to report those same symptoms in future cycles and will continue to say anxiety is the most severe.

However, a 1999 study found less symptom stability, especially for turmoil (agitation), fluid retention, somatic symptoms, and arousal symptoms. In general, researchers are less able to prove that symptoms like food cravings and breast tenderness consistently appear month after month and that they are equally severe in every cycle—and without consistency, treating PMS becomes more difficult.

Common Versus Uncommon Symptoms

Consistency aside, there is also the issue of the sheer range of PMS symptoms. Studies have documented some 200 different PMS symptoms, ranging from acne, asthma, vertigo, frequent urination, and rhinitis (inflammation of the nose), to heart palpitations, panic attacks, hot flashes, and in rare cases, even delusions and hallucinations. There are even some desirable PMS symptoms, although they are not widely discussed.

 Fact

Up to 15 percent of women experience positive or desirable symptoms during their premenstrual phase. These symptoms include increased activity, heightened sexuality, improved performance on certain types of tasks, and feeling energetic.

It would be difficult to divide the entire body of 200 symptoms into discrete types, especially since some symptoms are related to other health issues besides PMS. However, there are a number of PMS symptoms that are more common than others, and for this reason; it is valuable to look at them as types of PMS.

Type A (Anxiety)

If you suffer from anxiety, mood swings, irritability, and crying jags, you are in the great majority. Between 60 and 70 percent of women with PMS complain of these affective symptoms. The cyclical changes in estrogen and progesterone levels are thought to be responsible.

At the start of the luteal phase, the body has high levels of progesterone, which acts as an antidepressant and helps regulate the thyroid. But progesterone levels drop sharply as the menstrual cycle progresses. Estrogen can affect the levels of neurotransmitters, such as serotonin, in the brain and nervous system. As the levels of these hormones shift—sometimes up, sometimes down—in the second half of a woman's period, they can affect mood.

In addition, hormones affect how the thyroid functions, and low thyroid function can cause anxiety, among other symptoms, which makes it a possible culprit for Type A PMS.

Estrogen affects the body in many ways, such as:

- Helping maintain body temperature
- Perhaps delaying memory loss
- Stimulating breast development
- Helping regulate the liver's production of cholesterol
- Helping preserve bone density
- Stimulating the maturation of the ovaries, uterus, and vagina
- Helping regulate the menstrual cycle
- Affecting brain chemicals, including serotonin, dopamine, allopregnanolone, and endorphins, among others

Alternative, or complementary medicine, also blames poor liver function for the anxiety in this type of PMS because the liver is the organ that metabolizes, or breaks down, estrogen in the body. Often remedies include eliminating caffeine, alcohol, and nicotine, and "detoxifying" the liver with herbs such as milk thistle.

Essential

Alternative medicine, also known as complementary medicine, refers to practices that are not standard medical practice. These treatments can include chiropractic, homeopathy, herbal medicine, and acupuncture, as well as culturally based healing traditions, such as Chinese medicine. Most alternative treatments are not recognized as effective by the medical community, largely because there are few clinical studies supporting their efficacy.

Affective symptoms, as they're defined by conventional medicine, and Type A PMS are not the same thing! Affective PMS symptoms are a much broader category and include depression and food cravings, which are not considered part of Type A.

Type C (Carbohydrate or Cravings)

Some experts theorize that cravings may be an attempt by women to self-regulate the mood changes that accompany PMS. As women consume carbohydrates, they increase serotonin, which helps regulate mood and appetite. In other words, chocolate and French fries may improve the depression, tension, anger, confusion, sadness, and fatigue associated with PMS by altering brain chemicals.

Sometimes the symptoms of PMS are actually mimicking symptoms of hypoglycemia, or low blood sugar. Eating a carbohydrate-heavy meal or snack, such as a candy bar, causes blood sugar to rise. But those carbohydrates burn off quickly, and the person crashes. In an effort to raise energy levels once again, the person reaches for another carbohydrate-heavy food, thus precipitating another sugar rush, followed by its inevitable crash. This yo-yo pattern of highs and lows can lead to mood swings, headaches, and more cravings.

Low blood sugar has a number of symptoms that can be mistaken for PMS, such as:

- Anxiety
- Hunger
- Nervousness
- Nausea
- Sweating
- Coldness or clamminess
- Lethargy

One way to eliminate the highs and lows associated with both conditions is to eat several small meals (between five and six), rather than three large meals, to stave off hunger over the course of the day.

There is no such thing as a Type C PMS for conventional PMS experts. Symptoms such as food cravings and appetite changes are considered affective symptoms, part of the group of symptoms that impact mood. However, physicians do suggest diet (including supplements such as vitamin B6 and magnesium) or lifestyle changes as a first course of action in treating PMS. Type C PMS is a term used by alternative medicine, and suggested treatment may consist not only of dietary changes, but also of herbs such as dandelion, burdock, and milk thistle.

Type D (Depression)

Type D PMS includes depression, withdrawal, insomnia, forgetfulness, confusion, and lethargy. It is the down-in-the-dumps, I-can't-get-out-of-bed kind of PMS. This type is considered the least common and the most dangerous of all the types of PMS because women in this group are most likely to have the most severe and dangerous symptoms, such as suicidal thoughts. For a small majority, perhaps about 5 percent of women, this type of PMS becomes very severe and debilitating.

Type D PMS may appear similar to PMDD, but they are not the same. PMDD is a recognized mental health disorder that must be diagnosed by a physician or mental health expert.

Premenstrual dysphoric disorder is officially recognized as "a depressive disorder not otherwise specified." At least five of the eleven symptoms must be present for a diagnosis of PMDD.

In contrast, Type D is a loose constellation of symptoms. These symptoms are not consistent with how conventional medicine groups PMS symptoms. This type of PMS includes symptoms from three distinct clusters:

- **Affective/psychological:** Depression, withdrawal, lethargy
- **Somatic/physical:** Insomnia
- **Cognitive/performance:** Forgetfulness, confusion

There is also a danger of confusing Type D PMS with other mental health disorders, such as major depression.

Alternative medicine suggests several culprits for this type of PMS, including low levels of vitamin B, elevated tissue levels of lead, low estrogen/high progesterone, and low levels of neurotransmitters in the central nervous system. Some of these theories have no evidence, such as the theory that high levels of lead in the body cause PMS symptoms like muscle pains, fatigue, and headache. While lead poisoning can cause these symptoms and others, most cases in adults are the result of occupational exposure. PMS has not been proven to have any connection to lead levels.

Cyclical hormonal fluctuations do appear to trigger depressive symptoms, and as explained in Chapter 2, hormones fluctuate wildly during a woman's menstrual cycle. Low doses of vitamin B6 appear to alleviate PMS symptoms, but there is limited scientific evidence to support this practice. Alternative medicine also suggests natural progesterone to alleviate Type D PMS symptoms, while conventional medicine suggests antidepressants.

Type H (Hyperhydration)

In Type H PMS, women feel the effects of too much fluid in their bodies: bloating, weight gain, water retention, and breast tenderness. If you step on the scale and find you've suddenly gained six pounds, then you may be suffering from Type H PMS. Interestingly, constipation, which is more likely to be caused by dehydration rather than hyperhydration, is also considered symptomatic of Type H PMS. Possibly this is because constipation is a symptom of a slow-acting thyroid, a condition called hypothyroidism, which can also cause abdominal bloating. Up to 40 percent of women experience Type H PMS, which is considered the second, most common type of PMS behind Type A (Anxiety).

Fact

> Symptoms of hypothyroidism may mimic PMS and include bloating, malaise or fatigue, constipation, weight gain, and mood changes. It is believed that some women may actually be suffering from hypothyroidism when they believe they're suffering from PMS.

Prolactin's Role

Other theories about why some women tend to experience bloating and weight gain include elevated prolactin levels and low levels of magnesium and vitamin B6 (see Chapter 15). Elevated prolactin levels, which are known to cause amenorrhea or the condition of having no periods, may cause bloating, but research hasn't proven there is a definitive connection between high prolactin levels and PMS. For example, studies show that suppressing excess prolactin does not relieve bloating. Instead, many experts believe that thyroid abnormalities, which can cause bloating and are sometimes associated with elevated prolactin levels, may be responsible for this symptom.

Other Types of PMS

Don't get bogged down trying to understand your type of PMS. The popular practice of dividing PMS into distinct types can be confusing because there are differences in how these types are defined and labeled. For example, many resources will list four traditional types (anxiety, cravings, depression, and hyperhydration), while others will label them differently and add a fifth, headache.

The confusion arises chiefly when Type H refers not to hyperhydration, but to headache, and when the fifth category, Type B, is introduced. In this second Type H PMS, sufferers have a headache that is caused by increased swelling and water retention. Similarly, women with Type B PMS also retain water (here called bloating), but they also suffer from aggression, which is not included in any of the other categories.

Some resources also define two subgroups of PMS types: dysmenorrhea (painful periods), with back pain, nausea, and vomiting as the main symptoms; and acne, with pimples, oily skin, and oily hair as the main symptoms. However, the symptoms characterizing these subgroups may not have any relation to PMS at all.

Mixed Type

What if you suffer from Type A PMS during some months and from Type B in other months? Or what if you have symptoms from Type D, Type A and Type H? Are you the only one? How can you fit yourself into one of these categories? Perhaps you think you don't clearly understand all of the symptoms that define the different PMS types.

Relax! It's not you or what you understand or don't understand. The fault lies in the classification system. The truth is it's not perfect or even terribly accurate.

Many women experience symptoms that fit neatly into these predefined categories, but many other women do not. That's the nature of PMS: symptoms can shift over time, or from month to month—and you can easily feel symptoms from all the categories at once. In reality, many women have Type M (Mixed symptoms) PMS.

Using the Idea of Types

If you do plan to research and treat your PMS according to type, be careful and skeptical. Remember, these are popular, not medical, definitions. Categories shift, symptoms are grouped in multiple ways, and theories abound about the causes of the PMS symptoms. Even more important, treatments are everywhere, from milkweed and St. John's wort to antidepressants, and from an all-vegan diet to vitamin B6 supplementation. In many cases, women who use alternative therapies experience relief from PMS symptoms not because the treatments were shown to be objectively effective but because the women believed they worked. This experience, known as the placebo effect, is a well-known phenomenon. What works for you may not work for your friend or neighbor, and some of these treatments have little scientific evidence to support them.

CHAPTER 5

Physical Symptoms, Part One

BREAST TENDERNESS AND BLOATING are considered classic symptoms of PMS. As your body swells and aches every month, you might find that you're not only uncomfortable but also demoralized to see your weight escalate and embarrassed that you have to deal with gastrointestinal discomfort in addition to your period. This chapter will cover those classic PMS issues of bloating, weight gain, and gastrointestinal problems like constipation and diarrhea.

Breast Swelling and Tenderness

Breast pain is quite common in women—nearly 70 percent of women experience it at some point in their lives—and the symptom has long been associated with PMS. However, recent studies have shown that breast pain that regularly occurs before a woman's period, known as cyclical mastalgia, may not be a PMS symptom after all.

 Fact

The medical term for breast pain is mastalgia. Cyclical mastalgia or PMS-associated breast pain is pain that worsens in the premenstrual phase and is relieved when a woman gets her period.

When you have PMS, your breasts may feel full, engorged, achy, and painful to the touch; they may even feel bumpy or lumpy (although some women have naturally bumpy breasts). PMS-related breast pain and swelling can range from mild discomfort to severe pain, and one or both breasts may be affected. Approximately 8 to 10 percent of women experience moderate to severe breast pain before their periods. These symptoms typically peak just before the onset of the period and subside immediately after or during menses.

Some studies have shown that having breast pain before your period is not associated with PMS. A 1999 study by researchers at the Uniformed Services University of Health Sciences, Bethesda, Maryland, of thirty-two women with cyclical breast pain found that 82 percent of the women did not have PMS. A 2003 study in the journal *Obstetrics and Gynecology* found that women with breast pain might have wider milk ducts than women without pain. The more dilated the women's milk ducts were, the more pain they felt. These findings are leading many experts to rethink the causes of this classic PMS symptom.

 Alert

Some women have naturally lumpy breasts, a benign condition known as fibrocystic breasts (discussed later in this chapter). However, contact your doctor if you feel any unusual lumps or bumps in your breasts. Women should perform breast self-exams monthly!

The hormones estrogen and progesterone, which signal the milk-producing glands in the breasts to grow, are responsible for PMS-related pain and swelling. During the menstrual cycle, estrogen production increases and peaks just before mid-cycle. Estrogen causes the breast ducts to enlarge. Meanwhile progesterone, which peaks before your period, causes growth of the breast lobules. As areas around the glands expand with blood and other fluids to nourish the cells, they can cause nerve fibers to stretch, which results in a sense of pain.

In other words, if your breasts become painful during the luteal phase, it may have more to do with the physical structure of your breasts than with PMS. You simply have wider milk ducts that become more dilated in the second half of your cycle, and you may not even experience other PMS symptoms. For all practical purposes, if you feel cyclical breast pain during the second half of your cycle, you—and your doctor—probably consider it PMS.

L. Essential

Milk-producing breast tissue includes lobes, lobules, and ducts. Each breast has between fifteen and twenty lobes, which branch off into smaller lobules, and eventually into many tiny bulbs. Milk is produced in the bulbs and is carried by ducts into the nipples.

There are some risk factors for breast tenderness and swelling, including family history and diet, both of which are also risk factors for premenstrual syndrome in general. Caffeine, which contains mild stimulants called methylxanthines, and salt, which causes water-retention, are two common dietary offenders that can exacerbate swelling. Eliminating caffeine and salt, or at least cutting back on them, may improve your symptoms.

In many cases, doctors prescribe oral contraceptives to reduce breast pain and swelling. But for some women, oral contraceptives actually worsen these symptoms. If you are one of the women whose symptoms get worse while taking oral contraceptives, visit your doctor to see if you can take a different contraceptive pill.

Is it PMS?

Premenstrual syndrome may be the most common reason for breast tenderness, but it is not the only reason. First, is the pain cyclical? If so, do your breasts feel lumpy or bumpy during the premenstrual phase? If they do, you may have fibrocystic breasts. Contact your physician any time you feel any unusual lumps or bumps in your breasts.

Other possible causes of breast swelling and tenderness, besides PMS, include:

- Benign growths or cysts
- Pregnancy
- Fibrocystic breast condition
- Infection (if breastfeeding)
- Blocked milk duct (if breastfeeding)
- Muscle exertion
- Hormone treatments
- Oral contraceptives

Fibrocystic Breast Condition

Fibrocystic breast condition, which is related to hormonal changes during the menstrual cycle, is common among women between the ages of thirty and fifty; more than 50 percent of women have it. Typically, fibrocystic breasts feel lumpy and tender, and there are areas of thickening, with fluid-filled bumps called cysts, scar-like tissue, and pain. Although they can form anywhere in the breasts, lumps are usually felt along the upper and outer part of the breast, near the armpit. The lumps tend to be smooth and rounded, and they are not attached to other breast tissue.

⌷ Essential

Cysts are just one symptom of fibrocystic breasts. They form when the lymph system stores fluid in pockets of breast tissue. Eventually, fibrous tissue surrounds the fluid-filled pockets, thickens, and forms cysts.

Over the course of the menstrual cycle, these breast lumps may increase or decrease in size, and during the premenstrual phase, fibrocystic breasts are even more sensitive and tender. Symptoms usually abate with menopause, unless a woman is taking hormone replacement therapy.

The condition of having lumpy breasts used to be known as "fibrocystic breast disease." But since half of all women have lumpy breasts, most physicians now avoid the terms *disease* or even *condition*. Instead, lumpy breasts are more commonly referred to as fibrocystic breast condition, fibrocystic breast change, fibrocystic breast disease (favored by doctors in the past), or cystic disease.

Noncyclical Breast Pain

As the name implies, noncyclical breast pain is not tied to the menstrual cycle. Pain does not alternately worsen or improve over the course of the month but remains steady. In addition, women with this type of pain experience it in a specific area of the breast, such as the site of an injury or at the site of a breast biopsy.

 Fact

One cause of noncyclical pain is costochondritis, a type of arthritic pain at the breastbone, where the ribs and breastbone meet. Women with this condition often describe a burning sensation within the breast, although in reality the pain is coming from the bone. Costochondritis is caused by trauma or aging and can be exacerbated by poor posture.

Noncyclical breast pain most frequently occurs in women between the ages of forty and fifty. Part of this has to do with the aging process; some noncyclical pain is related to arthritis. Doctors have also found that physical stress and muscle exertion can cause breast pain. In this case, the chest-wall muscles hurt, but it is perceived as breast pain.

Noncyclical pain often subsides after one or two years and is not usually a sign of breast cancer, although you should consult your doctor about this condition.

Is the Pain Cyclical?

If you've confirmed that your breast pain is not related to pregnancy or infection, injury or stress, there are ways to manage it. For one, wear a good bra. Many times, moderate pain becomes excruciating because breasts have poor support. Second, treat the symptoms with over-the-counter pain relievers like Motrin or use hot and cold packs to manage pain and reduce swelling.

Here are a few tips to manage your aching breasts:

- **Wear a supportive bra.**
- **Exercise.** Sometimes moving around may help relieve the pain and reduce stress, which exacerbates pain.
- **Use ice to relieve swelling** and heat packs to ease pain.
- **Reduce salt and caffeine**, which anecdotal evidence suggests may relieve swelling.
- **Maintain a low-fat diet.** There is some anecdotal evidence that too much dietary fat causes breast pain and swelling.
- **Take vitamins B6, B1, and E** which have helped some women relieve pain. Some research shows that vitamin B6, in particular, helps relieve PMS symptoms, especially breast pain.
- **Try evening primrose.** This herb is believed to help reduce pain.

Bloating

Ugh. You know the feeling: your abdomen feels extended, tight, and swollen. You can't button or zip your skirt without strain. Sometimes even your hands and your feet feel swollen. Bloating is one of the more dispiriting symptoms of PMS; not only do you feel physically uncomfortable, but your clothes no longer fit.

PMS-related bloating is usually caused by water retention rather than an accumulation of intestinal gas, which may result after eating certain foods and from food allergies or as a result of swallowing excess air. But why do so many women feel bloated in the two weeks or so before their period? Experts believe it may have to do with the hormone aldosterone, which helps regulate the body's electrolyte balance.

⌐. Essential

Bloating is usually caused by poor or disorganized contractions of the upper intestine. The contractions move food and fluid along; if they are ineffective, bloating occurs.

Electrolytes, or salts as they are sometimes called, are minerals such as sodium, potassium, magnesium, and chloride that enable the body and heart to work properly. The kidneys control the amount of electrolytes in the body, and aldosterone regulates how the kidneys excrete these minerals.

During the second half of the menstrual cycle, after ovulation, aldosterone levels normally increase. This is also the time when estrogen levels are high. Estrogen intensifies the effects of aldosterone. This combination of high aldosterone and high estrogen causes fluid retention, which then leads to bloating.

Stress also increases aldosterone levels: when the body is stressed, the adrenal glands produce high levels of the stress hormones cortisone, hydrocortisone, and aldosterone.

Calcium and magnesium supplements have been shown to reduce bloating and fluid retention, as have diuretics. However, diuretics also eliminate potassium in the body, which can cause health problems.

Here are a few tips to help reduce bloating:

- Eat smaller, more frequent meals.
- Drink plenty of water.
- Reduce salt in your diet.
- Avoid foods that produce excess gas, such as beans, broccoli, peas, apricots, and bananas.
- Avoid dairy products if you are lactose intolerant.
- Try taking over-the-counter medications, such as Midol.

Fact

It may sound counterintuitive, but drinking water will actually reduce bloating. Water helps the kidneys function properly and flushes out toxins. You should drink between eight to ten 8-ounce glasses of water each day.

Weight Gain

The corollary to PMS-related bloating is often weight gain. A survey of more than 1,500 women found that about one in two experience bloating or weight gain during their cycle. In general, women with PMS report gaining anywhere between three to ten pounds during their premenstrual phase. The reasons for this are complicated.

First, some weight gain is genuinely caused by fluid retention, a common symptom of PMS. However, while women only gain a small amount of weight—between one and three pounds, for example—they are also plagued with all of the discomforts of bloating, such as feelings of skin tightness and heaviness. So how they experience their weight gain is exaggerated. These bloating-related discomforts may lead women to perceive they've gained more weight than they actually have, so the woman who has gained three pounds may feel as though she's gained ten pounds.

Weight gained as a result of fluid retention, or water weight, is usually temporary and the pounds come off as the woman gets her period or shortly thereafter.

Second, many women who have PMS or are diagnosed with PMS are older and as women age, their metabolism slows. A slower metabolism makes it harder to burn calories. Consequently, a poor diet, or PMS-induced cravings for sugary foods and other carbohydrates, may lead to quicker weight gain and an overall perception that weight gain is related to PMS, when it's actually related to eating habits.

Third, many women who suffer from PMS are prone to stress, and stress is a known trigger for overeating, which can lead to weight gain.

Finally, many of the foods that women crave while they're PMS-ing (e.g., chocolate, dairy, or salty snacks) can produce excess gas, cause the body to retain water, and cause bloating. Indulging in these foods ends up intensifying both the actual weight gain itself and the perception of that weight. It's a vicious cycle: stress, food cravings, and the hormonal processes that trigger bloating cause women to gain weight, eat more, and feel worse.

Upset Stomach

An upset stomach includes feelings of general discomfort, nausea, indigestion, flatulence, and heartburn. There are no statistics to determine exactly the number or percentage of women who regularly get an upset stomach in the two weeks or so before their periods, but upset stomach is common enough to be grouped among the thirty or so typical PMS symptoms by medical experts.

Diet, Stress, and Other Causes

An upset stomach can occur for many reasons; PMS is just one among them. Diet, stress, and side effects from medications are some of the most common causes, and each plays a role in PMS.

A 2006 survey showed that nearly one in three people who are stressed also had an upset stomach. The survey found that 32 percent of men and women who experienced stress also experienced frequent upset stomach or indigestion. Research has also shown that women prone to stress are also more likely to feel PMS symptoms.

Some medications used to treat PMS pain or insomnia list an upset stomach as one of their main side effects. Diets rich in gas-producing foods, poor in nutrients, high in fat, and low in fiber—typical for many women with PMS—often lead to an upset stomach.

Nonsteroidal Anti-inflammatory Drugs: The Chicken or the Egg?

Many women don't blink an eye when they pop a couple of Motrin or ibuprofen tablets to reduce PMS-associated pain. But one of the side effects of nonsteroidal anti-inflammatory drugs (NSAIDs), such as ibuprofen (Advil, Motrin IB) and naproxen sodium (Aleve), is upset stomach. If you're in the habit of taking NSAIDs to relieve premenstrual pain, you may actually be making some of your symptoms worse. Consider whether taking NSAIDs is causing or contributing to your upset stomach, or consider taking these drugs with an antacid.

Constipation

If you're constipated, you're not alone: according to a 1991 survey, more than 4 million Americans are frequently constipated. But constipation tends to be more common among pregnant women, older individuals, women following childbirth, following surgery, and PMS sufferers.

Essential

Constipation is defined as having bowel movements that are infrequent, with stools that are often hard and dry. However, what one individual considers infrequent, another considers normal. As a result, constipation is not determined by the number of bowel movements each day, but by the fact that they are reduced for a given person.

Normally, muscle contractions push food through the large intestine, and the colon absorbs water from food, forming waste products. If the contractions are slow or sluggish, food stays in the intestine longer and the colon absorbs more water, so stools are hard and dry.

Just as in upset stomach and bloating, constipation is tied to the withdrawal of progesterone in a woman's body. Progesterone is a smooth muscle relaxant, and the gut is a smooth muscle that moves fluid and food through the body by a series of contractions. As progesterone peaks in the premenstrual phase, it can weaken the contractions in the gut, resulting in bloating, indigestion, or constipation.

Diarrhea

You just can't win: First, you're constipated; then just days before your period you're running to the bathroom with diarrhea and cramps. What gives? This is another effect of the hormonal fluctuations that trigger your period.

After ovulation, when progesterone levels initially increase, they relax the smooth muscles in the body, such as the gut. The higher level of progesterone leads to slower muscle contractions, which can lead to bloating, indigestion, and constipation.

But after ovulation, estrogen levels drop and continue to fall. When the levels of both estrogen and progesterone fall, this can prompt cramping and diarrhea. Voilà! First, constipation, followed days later by diarrhea.

Prostaglandins

Another theory for PMS-related diarrhea has to do with prostaglandins, which are hormone-like substances that cause uterine contractions and cramps. Some studies have suggested that women with digestive problems complain of more severe PMS symptoms than those without digestive problems. Experts theorize the mechanisms involved in both menstrual and digestive problems are similar. Since prostaglandins prompt both uterine contractions and contractions of smooth muscle in the bowels, they are suspected in dysmenorrhea (painful periods), intestinal disorders such as irritable bowel syndrome, and some PMS symptoms such as cramps and diarrhea.

 Fact

Prostaglandins are a group of hormone-like substances produced in the cell membranes of body tissues. They may affect blood pressure, metabolism, and smooth muscle activity. Some prostaglandins reduce inflammation. Synthetic prostaglandins are used to induce labor.

Although uncomfortable, PMS-related diarrhea subsides with your period. In the meantime, do what you can to minimize symptoms: eat smaller meals, avoid foods that cause or intensify it, and use over-the-counter medications, if necessary. Here are some treatments for diarrhea you can try at home:

- Keep hydrated with sports drinks, which replace the body's electrolytes.
- Try the BRAT diet. Pediatricians and other physicians recommend this bland diet of bananas, rice, applesauce, and toast to ease diarrhea and nausea.
- Practice good hygiene to reduce the spread of germs.
- Try over-the-counter diarrhea medications.
- Consider taking evening primrose oil.

Evening Primrose Oil

Many alternative practitioners recommend evening primrose oil, or EPO, for PMS symptoms. This herbal remedy contains an essential fatty acid called gamma-linolenic acid (GLA) and is known as a prostaglandin precursor. Alternative medicine practitioners believe evening primrose oil is beneficial for many conditions, including irritable bowel syndrome; it is said to alleviate this condition in women during their premenstrual and menstrual phases. However, to date, there is insufficient medical evidence, in the form of controlled, systematic studies, to show that evening primrose oil reduces PMS symptoms.

While evening primrose oil has its proponents in alternative medicine, a number of clinical studies have found insufficient evidence to support its use or have concluded that it does not provide any relief for PMS. In contrast, one study from the Cedars-Sinai Integrative Medicine Medical Group, published in 2000 in the *Journal of the Pharmaceutical Association*, Washington, D.C., found that EPO was a reasonable treatment for some women with PMS.

CHAPTER 6

Oh, My Aching Head! Physical Symptoms, Part Two

FOR SOME WOMEN, GETTING PMS is not unlike getting the flu: their muscles, joints, and back ache; their head throbs and they're so exhausted they don't know what hit them. Do they feel lousy because they're going to get their period in a couple of weeks, or is it something else? The timing of symptoms is the greatest clue. If you feel achy and exhausted within that two-week window before your period, your hormones—and not a virus—may be to blame.

Headaches

Despite its catchall name, a headache is not uniform. It includes different types of pain—throbbing, pulsating, pounding, or tightness—and has many causes, from stress and eye strain, to hormonal shifts, high blood pressure, and illness. The premenstrual headache, experts believe, is caused by hormones, and women with this type of headache often describe having severe pain on one or both sides of the head that is accompanied by a host of other PMS symptoms, such as fatigue and joint pain. Headaches can be distinguished by the kind of pain they produce:

- **Tension:** Feels like a tightening, pressing, or a band-like sensation around the back of the head or neck
- **Migraine:** Throbbing pain, usually on one side of the head; may include nausea and sensitivity to light

- **Cluster:** Usually felt on one side of the head, can feel like a mild burning sensation; occurs in clusters, between one and four times a day, for periods that can last weeks or months
- **Hormone:** Severe pain on one or both sides of the head, during the luteal phase and accompanied by PMS symptoms, or during ovulation and menses and accompanied by nausea, vomiting, and aura
- **Rebound:** Nonspecific, generalized pain similar to tension headaches, caused by overuse of medications
- **Sinus:** Pain and pressure around the eyes, cheeks, and forehead; upper teeth may ache.
- **Secondary/Organic:** Can cause pain, confusion, and visual disturbances, or appear to change in pattern. (This type of headache is a symptom of another disorder or disease.)

Just because headaches are common doesn't mean men and women always get the same kinds of headaches or get them in equal numbers.

Essential

The most common types of headaches generally consist of acute pain, which means the pain is short-lived, localized, and fairly easily to identify. Headaches are one of the most common forms of pain in the United States.

For example, while nearly 80 percent of people experience a tension headache at some point in their lives, women are three times more likely than men to experience a migraine headache. In contrast, men are much more likely to get cluster headaches; 90 percent of people who get cluster headaches are male. In sheer numbers, however, migraine headaches are more prevalent; 29.5 million people get migraines, compared with the 1 million who get cluster headaches.

Headaches and Hormones

Headaches and hormones are related, but their connection is not entirely clear. Hormones, produced by the glands in the endocrine system, regulate a woman's menstrual cycle and appear to cause many PMS symptoms. Whether hormones are directly responsible for headaches, however, is still up for debate.

 Alert

Hormone headaches are not just a "female problem." Hormones induce the body's pain response, so in that sense all headaches are hormone headaches!

On the one hand, some evidence suggests the hormone-headache connection is strong. Some women experience headache at specific times during their monthly cycles (at ovulation, during the luteal phase, and during their periods). Women are more likely than men to get migraine headaches, and their migraines can disappear during pregnancy (a time of massive hormone changes) and may disappear or worsen after menopause (another time of massive hormonal change). On the other hand, some researchers believe that women who suffer from menstrual migraines (discussed later in this chapter) are predisposed to migraines and the fact that they get migraines during their period is actually more coincidental than causative.

However, the interplay of progesterone and estrogen, and their effect on the brain chemical serotonin, does play a role in how the brain perceives pain.

Research has shown that hormones—in particular, progesterone and estrogen—appear to regulate the brain's ability to suppress pain. This may explain why women are more likely than men to have disorders in which chronic and severe pain is a major symptom (e.g., fibromyalgia). When estrogen levels are high, such as during ovulation, the brain releases more endorphins, which inhibit the pain signals received by the brain. But when estrogen levels are low, as they are in the luteal (or premenstrual) phase of the menstrual cycle, the brain seems to produce fewer endorphins, resulting in more intense pain.

 Fact

> Although it does not have pain receptors and therefore cannot feel pain, the brain plays the greatest role in the perception of pain. It uses chemical messengers called neurotransmitters, such as endorphins, to transmit the sensation of pain to nerve cells throughout the body. The brain can also magnify or block the experience of pain.

Estrogen's Effect on Pain

In 2002, researchers at the University of Michigan conducted a study that demonstrated the effects of estrogen on pain perception. Fourteen men and fourteen women were given harmless but painful jaw injections and were then asked to rate their pain on a scale. Brain scans revealed that the women, who were in the early follicular phase of their cycles and had low estrogen levels, felt pain more intensely than the men. A subsequent study the following year looked at women in the early follicular phase, with low estrogen levels, and compared them while they wore an estrogen-releasing skin patch to mimic a later phase in their menstrual cycle when estrogen levels are higher. In the high estrogen phase, women reported their pain as less intense.

Serotonin

The neurotransmitter serotonin, which plays a big role in depression, is also thought to be the primary hormonal trigger for headaches. It appears to act as a filter for signals coming to the brain, screening out background or unwanted noise but admitting signals that demand attention. Studies have found that when serotonin levels are low, test subjects suffered headaches. But when they were injected with serotonin, the headaches disappeared. Estrogen increases production of serotonin and influences the way it binds to nerve cells.

Causes and Triggers

Although hormones play a big role in headaches, especially in premenstrual headaches and migraines, muscle tension, constricted blood vessels, and inflammation also cause pain. For example, tension headaches are caused by the tightening or tensing of facial and neck muscles (and sometimes by chemical or neurological imbalances), while cluster headaches, migraines, and fever headaches are caused by constricting blood vessels. Infections, strokes, and diseases can cause what are known as "inflammatory headaches" (sometimes referred to as organic or secondary headaches). Typically, these headaches are just a symptom of the underlying disorder.

The National Institute of Neurological Disorders and Stroke divides headaches into four categories, according to their causes:

- **Vascular:** Caused by constricted blood vessels; examples include migraine, fever headache (also known as toxic headache), and cluster headaches
- **Muscular:** Caused by muscle contraction; a prime example is the tension headache
- **Traction:** Caused by traction on intracranial structures; examples include pain produced by tumors, abscesses, or swelling
- **Inflammatory:** Caused by inflammation; examples include pain caused by sinus infection or meningitis

Headache Triggers

Stress, allergies, odors, medications, hormones, and certain foods are just some of the things that can trigger headaches—and interestingly, women are more vulnerable than men to all of them!

A 2002 study found that women who rely on over-the-counter pain relievers were anywhere from 4 percent to 17 percent more likely than men to get headaches triggered by stress, sinus allergies, foods, smells, spouses or children, and medications. The only thing men reported being more sensitive to was headache caused by cold beverages or ice cream. Twelve percent of men compared with 8 percent of women reported "brain freeze" headaches.

 Alert

Alcohol, caffeine, and salt, which can cause a number of PMS symptoms, are also headache triggers!

Migraines

As if it weren't enough that women get PMS headaches, they're also more vulnerable to migraines, a particularly painful type of headache that is sometimes accompanied by nausea, vomiting, and visual disturbances. Approximately 29.5 million people get migraines and nearly 70 percent of them are women. Overall, migraines are most common in people between the ages of fifteen and fifty-five, which also happens to be the span of time when most women menstruate.

So what causes migraines? Physiologically, migraines are caused by neural changes in the brain, but stress, diet, bright lights or noises, weather changes, a lack of food or sleep, and emotional distress are among the common triggers—and, of course, hormones.

Classic Versus Common

There are two forms of migraine: classic and common. A classic migraine includes visual symptoms (known as aura) that precede the headache by ten to thirty minutes. The person may see flashing lights or zigzag lines, may have blind spots, or may even lose vision for a time. There may also be sensory problems, such as disturbances in the sense of touch, taste, or smell. In common migraines, there is no aura. However, the person does have other migraine symptoms, such as nausea and vomiting.

Menstrual Migraines

Up to 60 percent of women who experience migraines get them during their periods or at ovulation. Known as menstrual migraines, these headaches appear to be caused by the dropping hormone levels that coincide with the period. As estrogen drops, so does the brain's ability to block pain sensation, which may trigger the migraine. Researchers have several theories on the causes of menstrual migraines:

- Falling estrogen levels trigger migraine headache by influencing levels or brain chemicals such as serotonin, dopamine, and endorphins.
- Serotonin, a known culprit in migraines, is affected by estrogen. As estrogen falls during the menstrual cycle, it's thought to disrupt the serotonin system and trigger a headache.
- Prostaglandins, which have been shown to cause migraines, trigger menstrual migraines when they are released in the bloodstream during a woman's period.

 Fact

An aura is a sensation of flashing lights or zigzag lines or a temporary loss of vision that often precedes a migraine headache. It is a warning that a migraine is about to occur. About 15 percent of people experience an aura before a migraine attack. The aura may last as long as an hour and will fade as the headache begins.

Ovulation Migraines

Another variation of menstrual migraine occurs at mid-cycle and is sometimes called the ovulation migraine. Fewer women report mid-cycle symptoms than migraine during their periods.

Given their timing, ovulation migraines appear hormonal. Although estrogen levels are high just before ovulation, women do experience rapid hormonal fluctuations. Experts believe these fluctuations disrupt the serotonin system and cause headaches. In other words, it's not the actual level of estrogen that triggers migraine but how the rapid shifts in estrogen impact serotonin. This same process is thought to underlie migraines that occur in some women who take birth control pills. According to the American Council for Headache Education, women who take oral contraceptives in which the doses and proportion of estrogen and progesterone vary tend to have migraine attacks during the week they take placebo pills, when hormone levels drop. This suggests that plummeting estrogen levels may trigger migraine. However, the exact nature of how oral contraceptives may or may not contribute to migraine is unknown.

 Alert

Your risk of migraine is highest in the first two days of your period. A 2000 study by researchers at the Headache Center at Thomas Jefferson University Hospital in Philadelphia found that women are twice as likely to experience a migraine without aura during the first two days of their cycle than at any other time of the month.

Oral Contraceptives

Oral contraceptives can both improve or worsen PMS symptoms, but in the case of migraines, many women find birth control pills actually trigger their migraines. A 2006 study of nearly 14,000 women in Norway found that migraines were 40 percent more common among women taking oral contraceptives. These women were also 20 percent more likely to suffer nonmigraine headaches.

Estrogen is thought to be the hormonal culprit in this case. Birth control pills can produce a fourfold increase in a woman's estrogen level. As a result, when women take their week's worth of placebo pills, they experience a rapid fall in estrogen, causing severe migraines during their "periods" (in the case of women taking birth control pills, this is actually withdrawal bleeding rather than an actual period). Some women find that taking continuous oral contraceptives, in which the hormonal dose remains constant throughout the cycle, can relieve their migraines.

Question

What are oral contraceptive placebo pills?
Placebo pills contain no medical ingredients, only inactive ingredients. Women take pills that contain hormones for three weeks and placebos for one week. The inactive pills cause the withdrawal bleeding that many women think of as their period.

Depression and Migraine

Until fairly recently, many doctors believed that migraine sufferers became depressed because their pain was so debilitating. However, research in the last decade has shown that the link between major depression and migraines is biological rather than psychological.

Researcher Naomi Breslau, Ph.D., a professor of psychiatry at Detroit's Henry Ford Health Sciences Center, conducted several studies on this subject. A 2001 study of more than 4,700 people between the ages of twenty-five and fifty-five found that people suffering from migraines had a greater chance of suffering from major depression than those not experiencing migraines. Similarly, people who suffered from major depression had a significantly higher chance of experiencing migraines than those who were not suffering from depression. In other words, the study suggests that depression did not simply arise from migraines, but instead the relationship between major depression and migraines worked in both directions.

Depression is already a key factor in PMS. Women who suffer from depression are more likely to suffer other types of PMS symptoms; research now confirms that they are also more likely to suffer from migraines.

Treating Menstrual Migraines

Usually, NSAIDs (nonsteroidal anti-inflammatory drugs) are the first line of defense against menstrual migraines. NSAIDs come in both over-the-counter (aspirin, ibuprofen, and naproxen) and prescription form (fenoprofen calcium, mefenamic acid). Sometimes, doctors may fight fire with fire by using the hormones to treat these hormone headaches. Triptans are the newest class of drug to treat menstrual migraines. These drugs chemically resemble serotonin so they are able to interact with the brain's serotonin system.

Migraine Therapies

Preventive treatment usually starts one to two days before the menstrual migraine and may be continued for five to ten days.

- **NSAIDs:** These drugs reduce inflammation by inhibiting an enzyme that makes prostaglandins. NSAIDs include aspirin, ibuprofen, naproxen sodium, fenoprofen calcium, and mefenamic acid.
- **Ergotamines:** These drugs are derived from an ergot fungus that constricts blood vessels.
- **Triptans:** These drugs reduce inflammation and constrict blood vessels by binding to serotonin receptors in the blood vessels and nerves.
- **Diuretics:** These drugs help reduce excess fluids in the body. Their effectiveness on migraine is anecdotal, rather than research-based.

- **Estrogen:** This hormone is usually given in synthetic form, as in oral contraceptives.

Alert

If you have significant headache pain that lasts more than a few days, your headaches wake up from sleep, you get frequent headaches with no known cause, or your headaches have changed in pattern or intensity, see a doctor for a medical diagnosis. A study of self-described sinus headache sufferers found that the vast majority had misdiagnosed themselves and were actually suffering from migraines.

Headache Diary

How can you tell if you get PMS headaches or menstrual migraines? The first step is to keep a headache diary, which will help you track the severity, frequency, and length of your pain and the possible triggers for your headache. It will also tell you if your headaches occur at ovulation, at menstruation, or during the luteal phase of your cycle. You can use a notebook to create your diary, or track your headaches on one of the several versions of headache diaries that are available on the Internet. Be sure to note the date and time your headache begins, its intensity, symptoms, and triggers, the kind of medication you use to treat it, and whether it resolves your pain. Include these questions in your headache diary:

- When did you start having headaches?
- How often do you get them?
- Is there a time of day or week they usually occur?
- Do you have pain on one or both sides of your head?
- What kind of pain is it? Throbbing? Pulsing?
- Do you have any other symptoms, such as vomiting or nausea?

- What triggers your headaches? Foods, activities, lights, noise, strong odors, smoke, stress, oversleeping?
- Does anyone else in your family suffer from headaches?
- How long do your headaches last?
- Do you have visual disturbances before your headaches?
- Do your headaches coincide with your menstrual cycle?

Joint and Muscle Pain

Aching muscles and stiff joints are fairly common PMS symptoms. One effect of the hormonal fluctuations that characterize the menstrual cycle is that they impact the levels of neurotransmitters such as endorphins in the body. Since endorphins increase feelings of pleasure and reduce pain, when their levels fall, pain is felt more intensely. Hence, muscles ache, joints are stiff, and there is a general feeling of being sore all over.

Of course, determining whether muscle and joint pain are really symptoms of PMS has to do with the timing of the symptoms. PMS is a constellation of very different symptoms that happen to occur in the second half of the menstrual cycle. If you have other PMS symptoms in addition to joint and muscle pain, and these symptoms occur reliably before your period, it's likely that you have PMS. However, there are disorders in which joint and muscle pain are major symptoms that are either intensified by PMS or mimic PMS. To get the best treatment, it's important to ascertain that your achiness is not caused by some condition other than PMS.

Fibromyalgia

In many ways, fibromyalgia looks like PMS: body pain, fatigue, stiffness, depression, and gastrointestinal pain and discomfort are among its major symptoms. Many people with fibromyalgia have sleep disorders, and like PMS, the condition is aggravated by stress. Also like PMS, fibromyalgia's symptoms can improve or worsen over time.

But unlike PMS, which combines physical, emotional, and psychological symptoms, the predominant feature of fibromyalgia is intense and chronic pain. Many fibromyalgia sufferers describe their pain as a deep muscular aching, or a throbbing or twitching pain. Their sleep is disturbed and their symptoms are often worse in the mornings. Like PMS, fibromyalgia is difficult to diagnose: it takes an average of five years for people to be properly diagnosed.

Question

What is fibromyalgia?
Fibromyalgia consists of pain in all four quadrants of the body for a minimum of three months, and pain in at least eleven of eighteen specified tender points when pressure is applied. It is often considered to be related to arthritis; although unlike arthritis, fibromyalgia does not cause inflammation or damage to the joints.

More women than men have fibromyalgia, and it usually strikes women between the ages of twenty-five and forty-five. In the early stages of the disorder, symptoms may appear together for only a few days at a time—another way in which this illness can mimic PMS.

Researchers believe that fibromyalgia is caused when the central nervous system abnormally processes sensory signals, which causes pain to be intensified. Other theories suggested that fibromyalgia is related to abnormally low levels of the stress hormone cortisol, which is produced by the adrenal gland. Women with PMS may have low cortisol levels as well. In addition, fibromyalgia patients also have low levels of serotonin (as do PMS sufferers) and increased substance P in the spinal cord (this is the protein substance in the spine that increases awareness of pain).

Alert

PMS and painful periods can also be symptoms of fibromyalgia! See your doctor if, in addition to severe PMS, you have symptoms consistent with fibromyalgia.

Although there is some overlap with PMS symptoms, fibromyalgia's major symptom is intense and chronic body pain. Here are some other key symptoms:

- Exhaustion/fatigue
- Sleep problems or insomnia
- Irritable bowel syndrome
- Anxiety
- Depression
- Dizziness
- Impaired memory
- Restless leg syndrome
- Skin sensitivity and rashes

Hypothyroidism

Hypothyroidism is the condition of having an underactive thyroid gland. People with hypothyroidism often have weight gain, dry skin, constipation, and joint pain, as well as muscle weakness, cramps, and stiffness. Since hormones are involved in the development and function of connective tissue (like that in joints), an imbalance in thyroid levels can lead to a thickening in the joints.

In general, hypothyroidism is not associated with PMS (only about 5 percent of women with PMS have hypothyroidism), but women with this condition may notice that their PMS improves if they receive thyroid hormone treatment.

Fact

> Hyperthyroidism, or Graves' disease, is an autoimmune disorder in which the thyroid is overactive. It can cause muscle weakness but not muscle or joint pain. Other symptoms include trouble sleeping, weight loss, irritability, heat sensitivity, a lighter menstrual flow, rapid heartbeat, and hand tremors. Contact your doctor if you suspect you have Graves' disease. Left untreated, this condition can lead to heart problems or other serious issues.

Backache

Attributing PMS-related back pain to a single cause is difficult. Back pain can be caused by any one of a number of factors or by a combination. For example, like joint and muscle pain, a PMS backache could be caused by the drop in the level of estrogen, which in turn prompts lower levels of endorphins and a sensation of greater pain. Or, depending on when during the premenstrual phase the pain occurs (for example, one or two days before a period), backache may be related to menstrual cramping. Stress and tension, both of which play big roles in PMS, may also prompt backache, and for some women, bloating exacerbates an aching back. So the issue becomes how to manage back pain. In general, over-the-counter medications, icing or warming the area, exercise, massage, and stretching will help relieve mild back pain. If backache is caused by inflammation, a simple dose of ibuprofen may be the answer, and heat or ice packs will help. For more severe pain, a doctor may prescribe muscle relaxants.

If you are sedentary, exercise will help relieve pain by making you more limber, strengthening your muscles, and helping relieve the stress and tension that often cause backache. Pilates, an exercise technique that improves strength and flexibility, may be especially helpful for backache because it focuses on working the core muscles, such as the abdominals, to support the spine and improve posture. Yoga can also provide relief.

Massage is a great way to relieve tension. For women with chronic back issues whose pain is worsened during PMS, chiropractic manipulation of the spine or acupressure may be very helpful.

 Alert

Studies have shown that chiropractic treatment is an effective, non-invasive treatment for back pain. Once dismissed by traditional medicine, chiropractic treatment has gained credibility among many doctors as research supporting its effectiveness has grown. Many insurers now cover chiropractic visits.

Here are a few strategies to manage back pain:

- Over-the-counter pain relievers
- Prescription muscle relaxants
- Chiropractic manipulation
- Exercise therapy, especially stretching
- Massage
- Acupuncture
- Yoga
- Pilates

Exhaustion

No doubt about it: PMS can be exhausting. Persistent physical pain or discomfort such as bloating or nausea, not to mention the emotional whipsawing that is so characteristic of PMS, is enough to exhaust anyone!

But fatigue and exhaustion in and of themselves are classic PMS symptoms. They are also associated with other conditions such as thyroid and adrenal dysfunction, depression, and fibromyalgia. As with backache, joint pain, muscle aches, and virtually any other PMS symptom, you have to pay attention to the times when you feel exhausted in order to determine if these are PMS-related symptoms.

PMS is a complex web of interrelated symptoms. Several PMS-related factors can cause exhaustion. Here are some questions that might help identify the cause of your fatigue:

- **Sleep problems:** Is your lack of energy related to a lack of sleep?
- **Depression:** Do you have other symptoms consistent with depression, such as feelings of hopelessness or difficulty concentrating?
- **Diet/nutritional deficiencies:** Is your diet balanced? Too little iron or vitamin B12 can cause exhaustion.
- **Stress:** Are you experiencing high levels of stress?

Hormonal Exhaustion?

Many practitioners of alternative medicine—such as nutritionists, naturopaths, and practitioners of Ayurvedic medicine and yoga—refer to "adrenal exhaustion" when describing a condition in which the adrenal glands, which produce the stress hormone adrenaline (also known as epinephrine), become overworked and cease to respond adequately. This condition then leads to fatigue, stress, and even depression.

Essentially, according to this theory, the adrenal glands are stressed to the point of malfunction, which degrades the body's ability to respond to stress.

 ## Question

What is hypoadrenia?
Hypoadrenia is a term used in alternative medicine to describe a reduction in adrenal activity. According to some alternative medical practitioners, doctors can't diagnose this condition because the blood tests used to test adrenal deficiency are not sensitive enough to detect adrenal fatigue.

Feeling Better

You don't have to be resigned to tiredness. Simple steps to feeling better include eating a balanced diet, getting enough rest, and reducing stress. In addition, treating physical symptoms such as bloating, diarrhea, headaches, or muscle pain will improve how you feel. Consult a doctor, however, if after you track your symptoms, you find that they correlate with conditions other than PMS, such as fibromyalgia or depression.

CHAPTER 7

Emotional Symptoms

THE EMOTIONAL UPHEAVALS OF PMS are so well known, they are the stuff of stereotypes. Who hasn't heard of the woman so moody she shifts from being irritated to weepy in the blink of an eye? Or the one who rages over the smallest incidents, her anger completely out of proportion to whatever set her off? It's a common stereotype, and many women have been in those shoes. But why does this emotional disorder happen to women, and what can be done to alleviate it?

Moodiness

Experiencing periods of moodiness is part of life. Women certainly don't have the corner on mood swings (although they often get blamed as if they do!). The tortured artist, the brooding musician, or the sensitive poet are all common images of moody people, usually men; but stereotypes often portray them in a positive or redeeming way.

In contrast, women with PMS are unpredictable, unprovoked, and out of line. The media often portrays these women as Dr. Jekyll and Mrs. Hyde, veering from nice to nasty at the drop of a dime. Knowing what happens in your body will help you understand your emotions, and why they so often seem uncontrollable during the premenstrual phase.

Moods and Your Body

Moods aren't just mental or emotional states; they create physical changes or responses in the body. Studies have also shown that emotions can affect the immune system.

- Fear causes heightened heartbeat, increased muscle tension, and an increased flinch response.
- Anger causes effects similar to fear, including heightened heartbeat and increased muscle tension.
- Sadness causes tightness in the eyes and throat and relaxation in the arms and legs.

Fluctuating Hormones, Fluctuating Moods?

Your periods can govern your moods, since the hormonal yo-yoing of the menstrual cycle has a demonstrated effect on emotions. Studies have shown, for example, that the hormones estrogen and progesterone intensify undesirable emotions, such as sadness, anxiety, and irritability in women with PMS. Other research suggests that some women are able to stabilize their mood swings even as their bodies are undergoing major hormonal shifts.

Essential

Neurologist David Silbersweig of Cornell University's Weill Medical College conducted a small study of twelve women with consistently steady moods during their cycle and found they had increased activity in the orbitofrontal cortex during the premenstrual phase of their cycle. The researchers believe this boost of brain activity may help women keep their emotions steady while their hormones fluctuate.

In addition, both perimenopausal and menopausal women can be treated with estrogen replacement therapy to reduce their mood symptoms, which illustrates the intimate relationship between hormones and mood. However, it's not yet clear why hormones cause mood swings, depression, irritability, or tension and why some women, like the ones in Dr. Silbersweig's study, are immune to these fluctuations.

Fact

A 2000 study of thirty-four women experiencing perimenopause (the early stages of menopause) found that estrogen significantly boosted mood in 80 percent of the women, while only 20 percent of women responded to a placebo pill. The estrogen improved feelings of sadness, irritability, and loss of enjoyment, but it did not improve sexual interest or assist with disturbed sleep.

The Female Brain

Scientists have devoted more time and money in the last decade to gender-based brain research to discover how men and women's brains operate. Researchers are also looking at what happens in women's brains during their menstrual cycle. One of the things that they are discovering is that there may be such a thing as the "female brain." For example, neuropsychiatrist Louann Brizendine, of San Francisco's Langley Porter Psychiatric Institute, argues that there are certain neurological reasons for women's behavior. She suggests that when hormones such as cortisol, estrogen, and dopamine flood a woman's brain, the woman becomes more stressed by emotional conflict compared to men.

 Question

Are emotions hardwired?
Some scientists say yes. Women have 11 percent more neurons in the brain that are devoted to emotions and memory. In addition, the amygdala, an almond-shaped cluster of neurons in the brain, acts differently in women and men. In women, the amygdala communicates with regions in the brain that help women respond to sensors inside their body. In men, the amygdala is more attuned to brain regions that respond to external stimuli.

Estrogen's Impact

Estrogen has multiple effects on the body and the brain: (1) it stabilizes mood; (2) it protects the heart from heart disease by reducing the body's total cholesterol level, while raising HDL or "good" cholesterol levels and lowering LDL or "bad" cholesterol levels; (3) it protects bones by preventing the release of calcium from bones into the bloodstream; and (4) it even prevents memory loss. Many of the mechanisms involved are interrelated, which makes it extremely difficult to link a single process to a given effect. Estrogen's other effects on the body include:

- Maintaining tissue elasticity
- Helping maintain vision (preventing cataracts and dry eyes, for example)
- Impacting the immune system by reducing the body's inflammatory response and increasing the production of antibodies that destroy bacteria and viruses
- Affecting the body's metabolism by impacting how carbohydrates and fats are metabolized
- Preventing vaginal atrophy

Estrogen has a cascade of effects on the brain and nervous system. For example, estrogen shares brain receptors with serotonin, which may explain why some women feel confused or foggy during PMS. It also binds the thyroid hormone, which means it influences the body's metabolism. Estrogen's effects on brain chemicals include:

- Increasing norepinephrine (involved in alertness, concentration, aggression)
- Decreasing dopamine (regulates movement, emotion, and mood)
- Having multiple effects on serotonin (affects emotions, behavior, and thought)
- Affecting blood tryptophan levels (the amino acid from which serotonin is made)

- Increasing endorphin levels in the brain and bloodstream (the body's natural painkillers)
- Protecting the acetylcholine systems (chemicals involved in cognition, motivation, attention)
- Having a complex relationship with DHEA (a neurosteroid with mood effects)

However, simply because estrogen's effects are demonstrable doesn't mean they're well understood. For example, although low estrogen levels are linked to depression, increasing estrogen will not necessarily cure depression. Hormone therapies, such as prescribing birth control pills to reduce PMS symptoms, may help some women, but researchers are not able to explain why they cannot help others.

 Alert

Estrogen may improve mood, but it poses substantial health risks! For example, in women who still have their uterus, taking estrogen alone can increase the risk of endometrial cancer (cancer of the lining of the uterus) because estrogen prevents menstruation, when endometrial cells are shed by the body. That's why birth control pills contain both estrogen and progesterone; the progesterone acts as a protectant from endometrial cancer because it causes the endometrial cells to be shed each month.

Irritability

It's almost a given that during PMS, one of the moods most women will experience will be extreme irritability. According to experts, irritability, tension, and dysphoria (a feeling of emotional or mental discomfort) are the most prominent and consistently described symptoms.

As your body's levels of estrogen fall, your moods become less stable. Plus, it's likely that your body will ache, your breasts will become sensitive or tender, you may feel nauseated or have diarrhea, and your clothes might feel more snug due to bloating. However, if your PMS-related irritability reaches the point where everyone needs to walk on eggshells around you, it may be worthwhile to consider examining whether there is anything in your lifestyle that is also contributing to your irritability. Some factors that increase irritability include:

- **Caffeine:** Whether in coffee, chocolate, tea, or soft drinks, caffeine will make you more jittery and irritable.
- **Carbohydrates:** Carbs provide the body with a quick sugar boost, but the sugar is rapidly metabolized, resulting in headaches, hunger, and crankiness.
- **Stress:** Too much stress will worsen your mood and cause irritability.
- **Sleep problems:** If you're not getting enough sleep you may be more irritable and cranky during the day.

Anger

Anger is a difficult enough emotion to deal with, but during the premenstrual phase, those feelings are often more intense and tougher to control. You're aggravated, you're moody, and you can blow at any time.

Most PMS experts believe these extreme feelings are part of the hormonal fallout of PMS, and many are using brain scans to look at how the brain is implicated in emotion. Experts also believe that anger is both a learned response (e.g., you are conditioned by your upbringing to respond with anger in certain situations) and an inherited trait. Studies have shown that some children are born irritable, touchy, and easily angered. Plus, our society tends to accept anxiety, depression, and other emotions but disapproves of anger. This makes it difficult for many people to express even normal anger and makes women who experience the emotional rollercoaster of PMS seem even more out of control.

Fact

Psychologists believe that some people have a low tolerance for frustration. These people get angrier if they are subjected to frustration, inconvenience, or annoyance than those with higher thresholds.

A Social Construct?

On the other end of the spectrum, there is a small contingent of scholars and researchers who believe that calling anger a PMS symptom is our society's way of dismissing a woman's feelings. Australian psychologist Jane Ussher is one of the best-known proponents of this theory.

To these scholars, PMS is an idea invented by our society in which women are told their feelings of anger and stress are biological rather than caused by other cultural issues. When women are told that their feelings are part of a disorder, the primary treatments are medical, but no one examines the real reasons so many women feel angry and irritated. This is a radical (and generally unpopular) point of view, but ultimately, researchers like Ussher believe that women are shortchanged by thinking their feelings are just part of the PMS phenomenon.

Managing Anger

If you feel like a hostage to your anger every month, you can take steps to manage it. There are multiple strategies, ranging from simple techniques you can try yourself to medication and therapy. Determining which one is right for you depends on the severity of your symptoms, as well as your treatment preferences. If your anger is mild (meaning, you don't find it interferes with your life), using simple strategies to manage your feelings is the easiest starting point. It's simple and low cost and generally involves identifying the stressors in your life and finding ways to relax.

Simple ways to manage your anger include:

- **Get to the root of your anger:** Identify the source of your anger (work, relationships, etc.) so you can deal with it appropriately.
- **Reduce stress:** Exercise, get a massage, or simply take time for yourself.
- **Take vitamins and calcium:** Improving your diet and increasing calcium has been shown to improve PMS symptoms dramatically.
- **Try relaxation therapy:** This includes visualizing relaxing experiences, telling yourself to breathe and picturing yourself relaxing.
- **See the funny side:** Humor can bring a more balanced perspective.
- **Reduce caffeine intake:** It can make you more irritable.

Therapy and Medications

If self-care doesn't solve the problem, then medication, therapy, or both may be the answer. Antidepressants are often prescribed for women who feel disabled by their feelings; they can't function in the workplace or their behavior interferes with their personal relationships. Prozac, one of the best-known antidepressants, not only reduces anxiety and depression but also has an anti-aggressive effect. Studies have shown SSRIs (selective serotonin reuptake inhibitors) to be effective in the treatment of PMS. On the other hand, therapy may be more appropriate if you are leery of taking medications or discover they leave you with unpleasant side effects.

Anger management is generally a system of therapeutic techniques that can help manage and control anger. This process can help you identify and avoid the things and events that trigger your anger.

Cognitive restructuring is another therapy to help manage anger. It allows you literally to change the way you think. Instead of flying off the handle, you tell yourself a more rational message, or you count to ten before saying something you'll regret.

Crying Spells

If you've got PMS, just seeing a dramatic movie, reading a sad or touching book, or being on the receiving end of an angry word can set off a crying spell. Whatever the circumstance, some women seem to cry a lot in the one or two weeks before their period for little or no apparent reason. Why do they do this? Experts believe that crying is an important way to relieve stress. This fits the PMS scenario perfectly: women with high stress levels are more likely to experience PMS symptoms, so crying spells are part of that stress reduction process. In addition, their moods are already unstable during PMS, so crying is easily triggered.

There's a lot more to crying than meets the eye. Experts believe that crying releases certain chemicals and hormones, which helps explain why most people feel better after crying. It restores the body's chemical and hormonal balance.

 Fact

Humans don't cry when running or engaging in other strenuous activities where rapid breathing is increased.

If you tend to cry during the PMS phase, you can take comfort, at the very least, in the fact that there are physiological reasons for your tears. Unless your crying is part of a wider spectrum of symptoms consistent with depression (in which case you should see a doctor) or your crying is socially inappropriate (e.g., at work), indulge the tears and you'll feel better.

Tension

For some women, PMS tension means tight muscles, an achy back or neck, or tension headaches. Others consider it stress or feeling jittery, anxious, or on edge. Whatever the case, tension is pretty common and may be caused by or related to any number of other PMS issues: high stress, a lack of sleep, physical discomfort, unstable moods, difficulty concentrating, or even depression. For example, you may be tense because you have PMS-related sleep problems or mood swings, or your tension may be the result of high stress levels, which is a risk factor for PMS.

The Causes of Tension and Pain

Physical pain and tension may—or may not— be related to hormones. For example, tension headaches appear to be related to low levels of estrogen (which impacts pain-reducing substances, such as serotonin) and muscle contractions (which are responsible for that tense feeling but may not even play a primary role in tension headache).

Magnesium may also play a role. It turns out that low levels of magnesium may trigger muscle tension, especially as related to tension headaches. A 2001 study by researchers at Brooklyn's Center for Cardiovascular and Muscle Research found that muscle tightness, tenderness, cramps, and strain were all related to tension headaches and to a magnesium deficiency. The study suggested that magnesium supplementation would be a "great benefit" in many situations.

Stress plays a role in pain and tension, both in a biological sense (stress hormones flood the body and produce physical effects, such as muscle contractions) and in a psychological sense (causing worry and anxiety).

High levels of estrogen in the body can cause anxiety. The week prior to the premenstrual period, when estrogen is high (estrogen peaks at about day fourteen of the cycle, then drops) and progesterone is low, may be riddled with anxiety and tension (remember, progesterone mediates the effects of estrogen).

Severe cases of tension or anxiety may require medication (e.g., antidepressants), but other milder forms of tension can be treated with the following:

- Over-the-counter pain relievers
- Massage
- Exercise
- Yoga
- Epsom salt bath (helps to relieve aches and pains)
- Elimination of caffeine and sugar
- Increased intake of magnesium

Positive PMS Symptoms

You could be part of the lucky percentage of women who report positive PMS symptoms. One 1999 study found that 66 percent of women say they have some positive premenstrual changes; those women most frequently reported increased sexual interest and enjoyment.

PMS is not all bad. These are some of the positive symptoms associated with PMS:

- The perception of having more attractive breasts
- More energy
- More creative ideas
- Increased sexual interest and enjoyment

Increased Sexual Desire

There are several documented times during the menstrual cycle when sexual desire seems to peak for certain women: at ovulation, in the follicular (the first half) phase, and in the late luteal phase. For example, many women feel a surge of sexual interest right before ovulation, which is when luteinizing hormone (which stimulates the growth and maturation of eggs) is at its peak. In this case, sexual desire is tied to the evolutionary desire to reproduce. Many women who do not experience PMS report their sexual interest peaks in the follicular phase, while women with PMS are more likely to report their interest peaks during the ovulatory phase, or late luteal phase.

CHAPTER 8

Psychological and Cognitive Symptoms

ONE OF THE MOST frustrating things about premenstrual syndrome is how it can throw you off balance psychologically. You feel anxious, confused, even depressed, but you're not quite sure why. It's as though a dark cloud hangs over you. You tell yourself it's your job, your family, your finances—and that very well may be the case, but there's something more that you just can't put your finger on. Then suddenly, you get your period and the skies miraculously clear. Welcome to PMS.

Am I Going Crazy?

The psychological symptoms of PMS don't always announce themselves like a guest ringing a doorbell. PMS-related changes in perceptions and behavior may be so subtle that you don't realize what's happening or aren't fully aware of the timing of your symptoms. Instead, you might dismiss your symptoms out of hand or ascribe them to other external causes.

Essential

Common psychological PMS symptoms include depression, anxiety, a feeling of helplessness, obsessive thoughts, the inability to concentrate, memory problems, and fuzzy thinking.

PMS is not only pervasive, it's also frequently mild. Of the millions of women who experience PMS symptoms at some point in their lives, only a small portion say it causes a noticeable change in their behavior and an even smaller number suffer severe symptoms. This means there are a great number of women whose anxiety, lack of energy, and fatigue are mild enough that they don't seek medical treatment for them. On the contrary, a great number of women aren't aware that their depression, anxiety, insomnia, and memory problems may be caused by PMS. In fact, it's not unusual for someone with PMS not even to realize she has it, until someone else—a husband, mother, sister, or friend—mentions the possibility. Remember, the majority of women are not officially diagnosed with PMS at all!

Essential

Of the 43 million to 55 million women who experience PMS symptoms annually, as many as 80 percent, or 34 million to 45 million women, experience mild symptoms that do not impact their behavior. These women are usually not diagnosed with PMS; they simply suffer from one or more PMS-related symptoms.

Ultimately, one of the best ways to determine if you have PMS-related anxiety or depression is to chart your symptoms and notice if they are cyclical. In fact, to be diagnosed as PMS, your symptoms must be tied to your menstrual cycle. When charting, note the severity of your symptoms. This will also help your doctor determine if you have PMS or some other condition. (Chapter 12 covers charting in more detail.)

Estrogen, Again

Why all the fuzzy-headedness during PMS? Once again, you can blame estrogen. Estrogen affects mood but also memory, attention, and language skills. For example, postmenopausal women, whose estrogen levels are low, often complain of memory and concentration problems, and the standard treatment used to relieve their symptoms is hormone replacement therapy. Indeed, a lot of what's known about estrogen's cognitive effects is the result of studies done on older, menopausal women.

 Fact

Estrogen enhances communication between neurons in the hippocampus, the area in the brain that plays an important role in verbal memory.

Women with PMS also complain of cognitive symptoms such as difficulty concentrating, but there is much less research to explain why this happens. In general, though, researchers believe that estrogen induces changes in how serotonin transmits, binds, and metabolizes in the regions of the brain associated with mood and cognition. What those changes are and their implications for treating PMS are not yet clear.

Is It Culture?

On the other hand, some researchers believe that women who experience negative cognitive or psychological PMS symptoms, such as depression and anxiety, do so because of their cultural perception of PMS rather than because of any physical processes or causes. In other words, women with anxiety, depression, sleep issues, or any other psychological, cognitive, emotional, or even physical symptoms feel worse because their culture tells them PMS is supposed to include those types of symptoms. For example, there is evidence that women report different PMS symptoms or different levels of severity in their symptoms depending on where they're from, their level of education, whether they're married, or if they have children. (See Chapter 3 for a more thorough discussion of the role of culture in PMS.)

Alert

A number of researchers have looked at how women's perceptions of PMS affect their reported symptoms. Evidence suggests there is some connection between how much women know about PMS and the degree to which they report negative symptoms.

There are also studies, such as the one conducted in 1977 by researcher D. N. Ruble, that suggest women report more negative symptoms if they believe they have PMS, even when they are in a different part of their menstrual cycle. Ruble told some women they were premenstrual and others that they were intermenstrual (that is, in the middle of their cycles), even though they were all intermenstrual. The women who believed they were premenstrual reported more negative symptoms. Another study conducted in 1999 found that women who watched a videotape describing PMS symptoms reported more severe symptoms after viewing it.

These studies suggest a few possibilities:

1. On some level, PMS sufferers buy into the idea that their pain is PMS-induced, instead of looking for other causes.
2. Once women understand there is a condition such as PMS, they pay more attention to symptoms they previously dismissed. In other words, knowing there is a genuine condition that includes their symptoms legitimizes their experience.
3. It is also possible that some women exaggerate their symptoms once they learn about PMS.

However, none of the studies linking PMS to culture or to theories about how women might exaggerate their symptoms based on their knowledge of PMS changes the fact that the anxiety and depression many women experience is real and affects their lives.

Anxiety

You know the feeling: sweaty palms, knots in your stomach, the feeling of being woozy or lightheaded. Anxiety is common—it can be caused by social situations, stress, medical conditions, or PMS. Our brain and nervous system regulate anxiety, and any disturbances, such as the complex interactions of hormonal fluctuations, brain chemicals, and behaviors that characterize the premenstrual phase, can increase a woman's anxiety levels.

However, if you suffer from unrelenting and intense anxiety, the kind that causes you to withdraw emotionally or prevents you from participating in normal day-to-day activities, you may suffer from an anxiety disorder.

Anxiety disorders can have multiple causes, including heredity, trauma, abuse, brain chemistry, low self-esteem, and even negative life experiences such as poverty. PMS can worsen the symptoms of an anxiety disorder. Talk to your doctor if you suspect you might have an anxiety disorder.

 Fact

Anxiety is a sense of apprehension or unease, often combined with fear and worry accompanied by physical sensations such as heart palpitations, chest pain, and shortness of breath. It can either be acute, with brief or intermittent episodes, or persistent and chronic. Acute anxiety can last for several hours or weeks.

The physical symptoms of anxiety include:

- Rapid or irregular heartbeat
- Nausea or a feeling of butterflies in the stomach
- Sweating
- Feeling cold or clammy
- Diarrhea, irritable bowel syndrome
- Headaches
- Dizziness or feeling lightheaded
- Shortness of breath
- Shaking, trembling, or twitching
- Insomnia
- Hot flashes or chills
- Rubbery legs
- Tingling in fingers or toes

Cognitive symptoms include:

- Fearfulness
- Worry
- Panic
- Dread
- Obsession
- Compulsion
- Nervousness
- Irritation
- Isolation from others
- Feeling intensely self-conscious or insecure
- Having a strong desire to escape

What Causes Anxiety?

Biology, genetics, and environment determine how people respond to stress. Anxiety is thought to be caused by a deficiency in serotonin (which modulates anxiety), and some people's genes simply make them more vulnerable to anxiety than others. In 1997, German scientists discovered there are variants in the gene that transports serotonin: one variant leads to more serotonin; the other variant leads to less. People whose genes make less serotonin are likelier to be anxious. Even with biology and genetics in play, environment plays a key role—people growing up in stressful circumstances, such as abuse or poverty, are more vulnerable to anxiety disorders, as are people who do not have self-confidence or who lack certain coping skills.

 Alert

Anxiety also has medical causes, which must be considered before a person can be diagnosed with an anxiety disorder. Two of the most frequently cited medical causes of anxiety are hyperthyroidism and Cushing's disease.

Anxiety Disorders

Anxiety during the premenstrual phase may be related to PMS, or it may be caused by a separate anxiety disorder. It's important to discern whether your anxious feelings are indeed PMS-related or if you need treatment for a specific disorder. There are five major types of anxiety disorders: generalized anxiety disorder (GAD), social anxiety disorder, panic attack disorder, post-traumatic stress disorder (PTSD), and obsessive-compulsive disorder (OCD). According to the National Institute of Mental Health, these disorders affect about 40 million people, age eighteen and older, the majority of them women.

Anxiety disorders combine physical and cognitive symptoms that can be aggravated by caffeine, drugs, or even over-the-counter cold medications. These disorders are usually treated with prescription medication, therapy, or both.

GAD: Constant Worry and Tension

Generalized anxiety disorder (GAD) is just one of the several anxiety disorders that may be confused with PMS-related anxiety. More than 6 million people in the United States have generalized anxiety disorder in any given year, and it usually affects more women than men. A person with GAD worries excessively, for periods up to six months or more, for no discernible reason and has symptoms such as restlessness, fatigue, irritability, and muscle tension.

Because this anxiety is not related to a particular traumatic event (as it is in PTSD) or marked by phobias or rituals, some women who believe they suffer from severe PMS-related anxiety may actually have generalized anxiety disorder.

The National Institute of Mental Health has a list of statements to help determine if you suffer from generalized anxiety disorder. If any of these statements applies to you over the past six months, you may have GAD.

- I never stop worrying about things big and small.
- I have headaches and other aches and pains for no reason.
- I am often tense and have trouble relaxing.
- I have trouble keeping my mind on one thing.
- I get crabby or grouchy.
- I have trouble falling asleep or staying asleep.
- I sweat and have hot flashes.
- I sometimes have a lump in my throat or feel like I need to throw up when I am worried.

 Fact

GAD can start in childhood, adolescence, or adulthood, but it first seems to strike women when they are in their twenties.

Social Anxiety Disorder

Many women with PMS are anxious about social situations, but relatively few will have social anxiety disorder. A person with social anxiety disorder worries about being embarrassed in public, but this condition goes beyond acute embarrassment, the kind where you want the floor to swallow you up. Social anxiety disorder can restrict a person's life by making it impossible to participate in social situations or maintain normal relationships. People with this condition worry about interactions others take for granted, such as:

- Being in a crowd
- Attending a party
- Eating and drinking in front of others
- Being at work
- Doing an activity in front of others, such as purchasing items at a store
- Shaking hands
- Being judged or evaluated by others

Social anxiety disorder, like other anxiety disorders, may be caused by chemical disturbances in the brain or may be genetic. A study by Harvard researcher Jerome Kagan, Ph.D., found that some shy infants have a higher-than-normal chance of developing social anxiety disorder as adolescents.

Panic Attacks/Panic Disorder

PMS-related anxiety can be severe, but unless you have panic disorder, you may not suffer the intense and often terrifying panic attacks that are symptoms of some anxiety disorders. Panic attacks are recurrent episodes of anxiety in which the person experiences chest pains, rapid breathing, dizziness, and tingling in fingers or toes and other physical symptoms. People with panic disorder develop a phobia of having panic attacks, which may lead them to avoid the situations and circumstances that they associate with the attacks, such as enclosed places.

Fact

According to the National Institute of Mental Health, panic disorder affects about 2.7 percent of people age eighteen and older in any given year. Panic attacks can be terrifying and can also lead to other complications, such as depression, phobias, or substance abuse.

Panic attacks can occur without warning; many people initially mistake a panic attack for a heart attack. There are three different types of panic attacks: spontaneous, specific, and situational. Spontaneous attacks come at any time regardless of the place or what the person is doing. Specific attacks are those related to specific feared situations or places, such as a public speaking engagement. Situational attacks are those in which a person is predisposed to have an attack in a certain situation or place even though they are not afraid of that particular place or situation. For example, a woman might be predisposed to having panic attacks in elevators, even though she is not actually afraid of elevators or enclosed places.

Post-Traumatic Stress Disorder

Post-traumatic stress disorder can be readily distinguished from PMS-related anxiety because it is brought on by a trauma of some kind, such as a serious accident, personal assaults such as rape, military combat, or terrorism incidents. People suffering from PTSD can have flashbacks of the traumatic event, have trouble sleeping, and feel isolated and detached; the condition frequently leads to problems in the person's personal life and substance abuse.

Obsessive-Compulsive Disorder

Most women who experience anxious feelings during PMS do not have the intrusive thoughts and compulsions that characterize obsessive-compulsive disorder. OCD is a condition in which a person experiences disturbing, unwanted thoughts and impulses to perform rituals (such as hand washing, counting, or cleaning) as a way to stop those thoughts. More than 3 million people have OCD, and it tends to run in families.

Anxiety Treatments

Anxiety disorders require medical attention and treatment. Less severe, PMS-induced anxiety can be managed by several simple strategies:

- Relax. Remove the stressors in your everyday life.
- Avoid caffeine.
- Visualize calming thoughts.
- Reduce noise. Turning down the television and stereo will have a calming effect.
- Exercise. This will help burn off pent-up energy and take the edge off your anxiety.

The three main ways of treating more complex anxiety disorders include cognitive therapy, behavioral therapy, and medication. Cognitive therapy helps identify the triggers of anxiety so that the person can remove them from his or her life. Behavioral therapy gradually exposes the person to the causes of anxiety in a controlled environment. It can also include using relaxation therapy to calm the patient. Finally, medications may include antianxiety medication, antidepressants, or beta-blockers, which regulate heartbeat.

Depression

Depression is a state of despondency, with symptoms such as fatigue, difficulty sleeping, and a loss of interest in everyday activity. Women are twice as likely as men to suffer from depression; 20 to 25 percent of women will experience a serious depressive episode at least once in their lives. Anxiety and depression seem to go hand in hand; research has shown that people with a major depressive episode are much more likely to suffer from an anxiety disorder, such as GAD.

Fact

In people with major depression, 85 percent also have generalized anxiety disorder, 35 percent have panic disorder, and 60 percent have feelings of anxiety.

Depression has many causes, including biology and external circumstances. For example, a family history or a medical condition may predispose a person to clinical depression, but events such as grief, job loss, divorce, living with chronic pain, and financial problems can also prompt depressive episodes. From a biological perspective, most experts believe depression is caused by low levels of the neurotransmitter serotonin.

Some common depression risk factors in women include:

- A family history of mood disorders
- Personal past history of mood disorders
- Using an oral contraceptive, especially one with high progesterone content
- Lower socioeconomic status
- Loss of a parent before age ten
- Sexual and physical abuse
- Using gonadotropin stimulants as part of infertility treatment
- Psychosocial stressors, such as job loss
- Losing a social support system, or the threat of such a loss
- Being a non-Caucasian woman
- Having financial problems
- Marital status (women in unhappy marriages, or who are separated or divorced)
- Having young children

The *DSM-IV*, the handbook published by the American Psychiatric Association and used to diagnose mental illness, lists depressive symptoms as the following:

- Depressed mood
- Feelings of hopelessness and worthlessness
- Suddenly feeling sad or tearful, with increased sensitivity to personal rejection
- Decreased interest in usual activities
- Lethargy or fatigue
- Marked lack of energy

Depression and anxiety exacerbate each other. A person who suffers from both depression and anxiety will have more severe symptoms than if he or she had each of the disorders separately.

 Alert

Depression and anxiety are risk factors for high blood pressure. Researchers from the Centers for Disease Control and Prevention followed more than 3,300 adults from the 1970s through the 1990s and found that adults (both male and female) with anxiety or depression had the highest odds of being treated for hypertension.

Treatments for Depression

Treatment for depression depends on how severe the illness is, ranging from self-help to drug therapy, psychotherapy, and even electroconvulsive therapy.

Drug therapies may include antidepressants such as SSRIs (selective serotonin reuptake inhibitors) or TCAs (tricyclic antidepressants), antipsychotic, and antianxiety medications. Therapy includes psychotherapy, light therapy, or electroconvulsive therapy (electric shock). Other options for people suffering from depression, promoted by alternative medical practitioners, include herbal treatment, exercise, and meditation, even aromatherapy, vitamins, and diet changes. (Chapters 3, 4, and 11 provide more information on depression, its connections to PMS, and treatment.)

Vagal Nerve Stimulation

Vagal nerve stimulation is used to help people whose depression resists other treatments. Doctors implant a small pacemaker in the brain, which sends tiny electrical pulses into the brain. First used on epileptic patients to eliminate seizures, the pacemakers also improved depressive symptoms. In a study of thirty patients conducted by John Rush, MD, at the University of Texas Southwestern Medical Center at Dallas, 40 percent showed a substantial decrease in depressive symptoms and 17 percent went into complete remission. However, this treatment remains controversial and a number of scientists question both the safety and effectiveness of the device used in this treatment.

Can You Repeat That?: Short-Term Memory Loss

Problems with short-term memory may be especially apparent during PMS. Short-term memory loss can be caused by hormones, stress, illness, and anxiety, all of which are factors in PMS.

 Fact

Short-term memory refers to the process when the brain stores information for a short period, generally between seconds and minutes in duration. Examples include remembering a phone number, address, or a random list or recent conversation. Experts believe short-term memory involves a temporary connection between neurons in the brain.

Memory and Estrogen

Estrogen's connection to Alzheimer's disease has opened new avenues of study into how it impacts memory in general. Estrogen appears to affect cells that are activated by serotonin and by acetylcholine, a neurotransmitter involved in learning and memory (Alzheimer's patients have reduced levels of both neurotransmitters), and facilitates how nerve cells communicate via these transmitters. In addition, there are multiple estrogen docking sites in the brain, including regions responsible for memory.

Although there is evidence that memory function declines as estrogen levels drop in aging women, at least one study found other factors besides aging impair memory function. The Seattle Midlife Women's Health Study, conducted at the University of Washington, followed 131 women in their early forties to early sixties and found that stress, perceived health, and depression were more closely related to perceived memory function than to the women's peri-menopausal stage or age.

Does PMS Improve Memory?

Although many women complain of problems concentrating or memory loss during PMS, researchers have found that memory varies across the menstrual cycle—and that certain types of memory might be improved during the luteal or PMS phase!

In a 2002 study, Pauline Maki, an associate professor of psychiatry and psychology at the University of Illinois, and two other colleagues, J. B. Rich and R. S. Rosenbaum, discovered that high levels of ovarian hormones such as estrogen and progesterone might inhibit the memory connections or associations that take place just before carrying out a task. Implicit memory (which does not require making a conscious effort to retrieve information, such as knowing how to walk or hold a pen) was better at the mid-luteal or PMS phase, while explicit memory (the kind that has to be consciously retrieved, such as remembering a book title) did not vary across the cycle. Maki and her colleagues speculate that estrogen may facilitate the automatic activation of verbal representations in memory.

Fact

Pauline Maki launched a study to test black cohosh and red clover as a possible alternative to standard hormone therapy. Black cohosh appears to bind to serotonin receptors, as antidepressants do, according to preliminary studies, while red clover contains compounds that are estrogen-like in function and structure.

Fuzzy Thinking

The foggy brain syndrome is another symptom of PMS. You feel as though you're slogging through mud, while everyone else is jogging along at a brisk clip. You just can't seem to think sharply, remember, or perform well.

For a long time, the medical establishment and even many women discounted this symptom, in part because "fuzzy thinking" is a subjective assessment of how any given individual functions. However, fuzzy thinking can also be a demonstrated effect of aging. Studies on menopausal women aged forty to sixty have shown that their memory and cognitive abilities improved after they underwent hormone replacement therapy. This has led researchers to begin accepting the idea that cognitive impairment may be real in many women and that it is somehow related to estrogen levels. Researchers think the findings on fuzzy thinking in older women may be applicable to women with PMS.

Difficulty Sleeping

Just as women are more likely to be depressed and anxious, they are also more likely to suffer from sleep problems. In fact, according to the National Sleep Foundation and other experts, sleep problems are twice as common in women as they are in men, and insomnia and other related symptoms may begin when a girl gets her period.

PMS-related sleep problems include difficulty falling asleep, staying asleep, or restless sleep. But why does it happen?

Sleep is regulated by the brain hormones and can be affected by external stimuli, such as temperature, noise, and sunlight. Levels of the sleep hormone melatonin are highest during the night, which promotes sleep. Though there is limited research on women and sleep, experts theorize that falling progesterone levels during PMS, or an increased sensitivity to hormonal fluctuations during the menstrual cycle, may cause problems during sleep. However, there aren't a lot of studies on women and sleep, or on PMS and sleep, to confirm these theories.

Essential

Sleep, depression, and PMS are linked: women are twice as likely as men to have insomnia, and insomnia is a risk factor for depression, which is highly correlated with PMS.

In addition, women with PMS often suffer from conditions or symptoms that cause sleep problems. For example, mood disorders, which are known to cause sleep problems, are a risk factor for PMS, and high stress levels, also correlated with PMS, can cause problems with sleep. In other words, mood disorders and high stress levels are associated with PMS.

PMS Disrupts Sleep

A 1998 telephone survey by the National Sleep Foundation found that 70 percent of women reported that their sleep patterns were affected by premenstrual symptoms such as breast tenderness, bloating, and headaches. Young women without significant PMS complaints reported poor sleep quality in the three to six days before their periods and during four days of their menstrual cycles. It's common, in other words, to have trouble sleeping because of other PMS symptoms, and PMS does not have to be severe for sleep problems to occur. The study also found that women in the luteal phase of the menstrual cycle have elevated body temperature during sleep, women on oral contraceptives have reduced periods of deep sleep, and women with dysmenorrhea (painful periods) have significantly disturbed sleep quality before their periods.

There are simple steps to take to improve your sleep, such as changing your diet to avoid caffeine and large meals before bed and avoiding naps during the day. Other tips for better sleep include:

- Establishing a regular bedtime routine
- Keeping your bedroom as dark as possible
- Unwinding before bedtime (Try relaxation techniques such as meditation.)
- Lowering the temperature (but keep it comfortable) of the room to promote deep sleep
- Seeing the sun (Get adequate exposure to natural light during the day.)
- Using the bedroom for sleeping and sexual activity only; not work or television

CHAPTER 9

Questions to Ask Your Doctor

YOU PROBABLY DIDN'T EXPECT to become a detective, but with PMS, more often than not, that's exactly what you have to be: a health detective who is attuned to your body, your symptoms, and their timing. You should also work in partnership with your doctor to discover if there are other health conditions or elements in your life that might be causing or worsening your physical, emotional, or psychological symptoms.

Play the Detective

You may think PMS is common and recognizable, but don't be misled by so-called typical symptoms. They all have more than one possible culprit.

Do you have breast pain and tenderness? Sure, it may be PMS, but it can also be fibrocystic breasts, pregnancy, too much sodium in your diet, or even muscle strain. Bloating and nausea? It could be irritable bowel syndrome, lactose intolerance, or the stomach flu. Do you suffer from raging headaches? Maybe they're caused by bad posture, too much time spent staring at a computer, carbohydrate binges, or over-reliance on pain relievers.

Additionally, our habits and health conditions often work in concert so that PMS symptoms can become more severe and more extensive, but their exact causes can be tough to pin down. A stressful job may cause not only physical pain (headache and backache, for example), but also drive you to eat poorly and not exercise, so that you're bloated, constipated, have low energy, and generally feel unwell—on top of having PMS! Severe PMS can make you depressed and having depression exacerbates PMS symptoms. If you're older, what you think is PMS might actually be perimenopause.

If you're not entirely sure you have PMS, something else, or both, here are some things to think about:

- **Do the people in your life say you have PMS?** If the symptoms are mild and there are other issues in your life that cause you stress or pain, you may not even realize your symptoms are cyclical. However, your family or friends might give you a better perspective.
- **Does your weight fluctuate every month?**
- **Are you sleeping well?** Sleep problems are one sign of PMS.
- **Have your periods been regular, or have you missed a cycle recently?** Irregular cycles for older women are one sign of perimenopause.
- **At what point in your cycle do your symptoms appear? At ovulation?** Just before your period?
- **Do your symptoms abate after your period?**
- **Are your symptoms primarily physical, emotional, or cognitive?** Do you have a combination of symptoms?
- **Do you have the same symptoms every month, or do they vary from month to month?** PMS symptoms can fluctuate from cycle to cycle, but if your symptoms suddenly shift, it could indicate another cause.
- **How long have you suspected PMS?**
- **Has your PMS gotten worse over time?**

Answering these questions should help you clarify your experience and prove useful in confirming whether you have PMS.

Going to the Doctor
Your family physician or gynecologist is a good first point of contact. He or she can help you decipher what's going on with your body,

identify possible causes, and suggest ways to relieve pain. He or she will also be able to refer you to other experts for further help if necessary. However, it helps to go to the doctor prepared.

You should expect not only to ask questions but to answer them as well. If you have severe PMS symptoms and want treatment at the time of your first visit, you may be in for an unpleasant surprise. Medical doctors will only diagnose PMS if you chart your symptoms for two to three months, and their first course of action is usually to prescribe self-care, such as exercise or diet changes.

PMS is diagnosed when symptoms occur regularly and in the late luteal phase of a woman's cycle. The American College of Obstetrics and Gynecology uses the following diagnostic criteria:

- At least one affective or somatic symptom during the five days before menses in each of the three previous cycles (Affective symptoms include depression, angry outbursts, irritability, anxiety, confusion, social withdrawal; somatic symptoms include breast tenderness, abdominal bloating, headache, swelling of extremities)
- Symptoms are relieved from days four through thirteen of the menstrual cycle (Day One is the first day of bleeding.)

If you haven't begun to chart your symptoms or don't keep track of your periods, now is the time to start. (Chapter 13 explains how to keep both menstrual and PMS diaries and provides examples of what they might look like.)

 Alert

Some doctors may have you rate your symptoms on a scale of one to ten, so they can better understand the severity of your pain and determine a proper diagnosis. Consider incorporating this information into your PMS diary.

Once you see your medical provider, use the appointment time to initiate a conversation about PMS: describe the symptoms, your medical history, and any stressors that impact your life. When talking to your doctor, here are some of the questions you might want to ask:

- Are my symptoms consistent with PMS? (What you consider a PMS symptom may not be, or it may be caused by some other condition.)
- Can stress be causing my symptoms? (Be prepared to describe your symptoms, as well as to describe how often and how severely you experience them, and expect to list the things, events, or people in your life that cause you stress.)
- Is it my diet? (The kinds of food you eat may cause mood swings and bloating.)
- Is it a nutritional deficiency? (Calcium, magnesium, and vitamins D and E have all been implicated in PMS. Keep a food diary or describe your diet to your physician.)
- What treatments are available?
- Will birth control pills help? (For some women, oral contraceptives relieve PMS symptoms; other women experience worsening symptoms.)
- Can I take over-the-counter pain relievers?
- How will they interact with my medications?

Essential

Eating a diet rich in vitamin D and calcium may decrease your chance of developing PMS. A 2005 study in the *Archives of Internal Medicine* found that women who ate at least 1,200 milligrams of calcium and 400 IU (international units) of vitamin D every day had a 40 percent lower risk of developing PMS.

Your doctor will want to know when in your cycle your symptoms appear, when they disappear, and when they are mildest or most severe. The more detail you can provide, the better your chances are of getting effective treatment. In addition, since some PMS-like symptoms may be related to irregular periods, it's important to know if you ovulate regularly. (Chapter 13 covers how to keep menstrual and PMS diaries.)

Is It My Thyroid?

Thyroid disease and PMS may be mistaken for each other. Women with hypothyroidism, the most common type of thyroid disease, often feel exhausted, have muscle and joint pains or aches, suffer from depression and other mood changes, gain weight, and are bloated. Thyroid disease also often affects the menstrual cycle, triggering or delaying menstruation, affecting menstrual flow, increasing the frequency of periods, or making them stop for long periods.

 Fact

The thyroid, a butterfly-shaped gland located just below the Adam's apple, regulates the body's metabolism. Thyroid hormone levels that are too high make people feel anxious, while thyroid hormone levels that are too low cause people to feel depressed and sluggish.

Thyroid disease is fairly common, and it affects more women than men. Nearly 10 percent of women have thyroid disease, compared with about 5 percent of men. It takes two major forms: hypothyroidism, in which an underactive thyroid produces too little hormone, and hyperthyroidism, in which an overactive thyroid produces too much hormone. Both forms usually develop early in life, but older women (especially those entering menopause) and women who have recently been pregnant face increased risk. For reasons that are not entirely clear, about 10 percent of women will develop a thyroid disorder after pregnancy.

Symptoms and Causes

Thyroid disease can be caused by thyroid removal (such as in the case of cancer or infection), by an autoimmune disease or an autoimmune reaction (in which the body produces antibodies against the thyroid gland); and by certain foods and medications. For example, hyperthyroidism, in which the metabolism is accelerated, is most frequently caused by Graves' disease, an autoimmune disease that is common in some women, especially older women.

 Alert

Goiters, or enlarged thyroids, are a highly visible symptom of Graves' disease, which causes an overproduction of thyroid hormone. However, most goiters are actually caused by an underactive thyroid gland.

The symptoms of hypothyroidism relate to a slowing of the metabolism and include the following:

- Weight gain
- Constipation
- Muscle cramps
- Confusion
- A swollen or puffy face
- Bloating
- Coarse and dry hair
- Thinning eyebrows
- Depression
- Carpal tunnel syndrome, hand tingling or pain
- Goiter (swelling in the neck area)
- Increased menstrual flow

Symptoms of hyperthyroidism, which causes an accelerated metabolism, include the following:

- Nervousness/anxiety
- Fatigue
- Heart palpitations
- Trembling gaze
- Insomnia
- Increased bowel movements
- Weight loss
- Absent or light menstrual periods

Thyroid Diseases and Menstruation

Thyroid disease can either delay puberty in girls or cause them to get their periods very early (usually before age nine). In women, hypothyroidism may cause frequent, heavy periods that sometimes lead to anemia, while hyperthyroidism can decrease menstrual flow and may even cause periods to end. In addition, both forms of thyroid disease have been linked to mood disorders and decreased sexual interest.

Essential

Since some symptoms of hypothyroidism mimic those of pregnancy, such as fatigue and weight gain, pregnant women may have thyroid disease and not even know it. In addition, some pregnant women develop a thyroid inflammation known as postpartum thyroiditis shortly after giving birth.

If you complain of PMS symptoms, your doctor may test your thyroid function. These tests measure levels of the hormones T4, T3, and TSH in your blood to evaluate how well your thyroid gland is working.

Women with thyroid disease may experience menopause before age forty. In addition, symptoms of hyperthyroidism, such as hot flashes, absent periods, insomnia and mood swings, may be confused with menopause. Once the thyroid disease is treated, normal menstrual cycles return and a normal timeline for menopause is restored.

Treating PMS, Treating Thyroid Disease

Although symptoms of thyroid disease often mimic PMS (depending on the thyroid disease, it can refer to high or low levels of the hormone), the thyroid hormone does not appear to be linked to premenstrual syndrome, except for the small percentage of women with both conditions. Medical doctors do not treat PMS with thyroid hormones. In contrast, many alternative medicine practitioners see a connection between the thyroid and PMS and often treat both thyroid disease and PMS with progesterone (which regulates the thyroid gland).

Thyroid disorders are treated with anti-thyroid drugs, radioactive iodine-131, or, in rare cases, thyroid surgery, depending on the form of the disease. Women who develop postpartum thyroiditis are treated with a drug called levothyroxine, a synthetic thyroid hormone. These treatments are usually very successful. However, since diet is one significant cause of thyroid disease, it's important that to avoid eating large quantities of goiter-producing foods, such as cabbage, broccoli and pears, and it is recommended to eat them raw.

 Fact

Some foods decrease thyroid hormone production and increase your chance of developing a goiter. These foods, known as "goitrogenics," include mustard greens, Brussels sprouts, turnips, rutabaga, kale, cauliflower, radishes, African cassava, peaches, strawberries, millet (a kind of grain), corn, and potatoes. Cooking these foods seems to break down the enzymes that affect the thyroid.

Are the Symptoms Related to Other Medications?

Your fuzzy-headedness, tender breasts, mood swings, and bloating may not be PMS at all. Rather, they may be side effects of other medications. For example, antidepressants, oral contraceptives, and drugs used to treat infertility can mimic PMS symptoms. So can synthetic progesterone, which is used in hormone replacement therapy, and other drugs that are used to treat endometriosis.

 Alert

> Be an active and alert patient. Note the medications you take, the dosages, and their effects as part of your PMS diary.

Be sure to disclose fully to your physician any other medications you're taking, whether they are prescription drugs, over-the-counter pain-relievers, vitamins, diuretics, or herbal supplements, so that he or she can take that information into account when recommending treatments. Your doctor may relieve your symptoms by suggesting other medications for your health conditions or disease, or at least, he or she will consider how PMS treatment will interact with the drugs you're currently taking.

Is It Perimenopause?

The transitional phase between normal fertility and menopause is known as perimenopause. During this time, levels of estrogen and progesterone drop, and periods become irregular—sometimes clustering and coming more frequently, then disappearing for months before starting again. Perimenopause can last anywhere from a few months to as long as a decade, and how long it lasts depends to some degree on family history, although on average it lasts about four years.

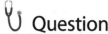

Essential

> The average age for the onset of perimenopause is forty-eight, but estrogen levels start to change a decade earlier, when a woman is about thirty-eight. Perimenopause can start for women who are in their mid-thirties, although those cases are highly unusual. Also women who smoke tend to go through perimenopause one to two years earlier than other women.

Perimenopause also usually causes a number of cognitive and physical symptoms, such as forgetfulness, hot flashes (sometimes more intense than those of menopause), decreased sexual interest, decreased energy, mood swings, fuzzy thinking, heart palpitations, heartburn, vaginal dryness, urinary problems (incontinence, more frequent urinary tract infections, etc.), and sleep problems.

Question

> **What causes hot flashes?**
> The decline in estrogen levels affects the hypothalamus, a small structure at the base of the brain that serves as your body's thermostat. If the brain believes your body temperature is too hot, it will send blood from the organs to the surface in an effort to cool off. Your heart beats faster, your blood vessels dilate, and you sweat. A woman's skin temperature can rise as much as 6°C during a hot flash!

Doctors used to determine if women were in menopause, or the absence of periods for twelve months, by testing the levels of follicle-stimulating hormone in their blood. However, studies have shown that FSH levels fluctuate dramatically from month to month, until a woman's periods have stopped. Now, menopause has been defined by not having periods for a full year, but very high levels of FSH, which are used as an indicator of ovarian reserve, have recently become indicative of menopause.

Hormones for Perimenopause

Just as is the case for PMS, your doctor might prescribe oral contraceptives to manage the symptoms of perimenopause (which would both restore regular menstrual cycles and reduce hot flashes). Other options include hormone skin patches and selective serotonin reuptake inhibitors (SSRIs), both of which reduce hot flashes. You should also modify your diet to avoid foods that intensify hot flashes, such as caffeine, alcohol, and spicy foods.

 Alert

Low libido may be caused by medication not perimenopause. Decreased sexual interest, a fairly common complaint of older women undergoing perimenopause, can also be caused by certain medications, such as drugs for high blood pressure and depression. Check with your doctor if you experience this symptom to rule out other causes.

Should I Be Taking Something?

Whether you're a candidate for medication depends on the severity of your symptoms, your tolerance for certain drugs (and their potential side effects), and your preferences. The side effects of some medications may leave you feeling worse than plain PMS, but if your PMS significantly disrupts your life, medication may be the best answer.

Most physicians will suggest you alter your lifestyle before they prescribe drugs. This is the point at which you should cut back on caffeine, alcohol, sodium, and sugar and increase exercise. In addition, if you are open to complementary medicine, such as chiropractic, acupuncture, yoga or herbal supplements, you may find these approaches provide ample relief. However, proceed with caution if you decide to pursue complementary or alternative medicine, as some commonly advocated forms of alternative therapy for PMS, such as evening primrose oil and progesterone creams, have been shown to provide no more relief than placebos.

Drug Treatments

Medications for PMS range from over-the-counter anti-inflammatory drugs and diuretics to birth control pills, hormone treatments, antidepressants, and antianxiety drugs. Which ones you take depends on which PMS symptoms are most severe.

Remember, before you consider taking any medication, ask your doctor the following questions:

- How effective is this medication?
- What are the potential side effects?
- How will this drug interact with the medications and supplements I'm currently taking?
- How long before I feel the effects?
- When do the side effects develop? How can I tell?
- Are there any things I should avoid while taking this drug?

Nonsteroidal anti-inflammatory drugs (NSAIDs)

Nonsteroidal anti-inflammatory drugs include over-the-counter versions such as aspirin and ibuprofen, as well as prescription versions. These drugs reduce inflammation by reducing prostaglandins (implicated in PMS) and are used to alleviate breast pain, headache, and menstrual cramps. However, prostaglandins also affect the stomach, so side effects include indigestion and heartburn, which means these drugs are not recommended for people with ulcers. (Some prescription versions have components that reduce the risk of ulceration.)

Diuretics

Diuretics, sometimes known as "water pills," force the body to eliminate fluid through urination and are used for bloating, swelling and PMS-related weight gain. (They are also used to treat high blood pressure, congestive heart failure, and glaucoma.) Diuretics are available both in over-the-counter versions, such as Pamprin and Midol, as well as in prescription form (such as spironolactone and metolazone).

 ## Fact

Caffeine, alcohol, and cranberry juice are weak diuretics. Vitamin B6 is a natural diuretic.

Oral Contraceptives

Most oral contraceptives contain two hormone compounds, estrogen and progestin, and reduce many PMS symptoms, except for some mood symptoms. One brand of pill in particular, Yasmin, which contains estrogen and drospirenone, has been shown to have specific PMS-reducing effects, including reducing bloating and appetite changes. Another oral contraceptive containing only progestin is usually prescribed for women who suffer severe headaches or high blood pressure, and for women who are breastfeeding. Progestin-only pills do not block ovulation and must be taken at the same time each day.

 ## Alert

A 2002 analysis did not find any benefit from progestin-only contraceptives for women with PMS, however a 2002 British study found that progestin-only contraceptives were the most commonly prescribed for PMS symptoms. Check with your doctor to make sure you're taking the right formulation.

Hormone Treatments

Hormones such as nafarelin (Synarel), leuprolide (Lupron), and danazol (Danocrine) are used to stop ovulation (and your periods) by blocking GnRH (gonadotropin-releasing hormone), the hormone that stimulates the ovaries and starts the menstrual cycle, because when you don't ovulate, you can't get PMS. Up to half the women who receive hormone treatment get relief for their PMS symptoms. However, hormone treatments have their drawbacks. For one, they cause an artificial menopause, which has its own complications, such as osteoporosis. In addition, danazol may increase certain fat levels in the blood, so its not recommended for women with high cholesterol.

Progesterone

Progesterone therapy is quite popular in alternative medicine and even among some physicians, but studies have shown it provides no relief for PMS symptoms. The treatment is also not approved by the Food and Drug Administration. However, it is still prescribed by some doctors. Many alternative practitioners also promote progesterone creams or lotions.

Selective Serotonin Reuptake Inhibitors (SSRIs)

These are usually the drug of choice for PMS-related depression, irritability, and anxiety; up to 60 percent of women experience relief while taking them. Side effects include drowsiness, nausea, and jitteriness. Women who decide to stop taking SSRIs must reduce their dosages very gradually to avoid side effects. (Chapter 18 has more information on SSRIs.)

Antidepressants

Antidepressants such as fluoxetine hydrochloride (Sarafem or Prozac), sertraline (Zoloft), and paroxetine (Paxil) work by increasing serotonin activity in the brain. But they can cause serious side effects, such as nervousness, weight loss, uncontrollable hand shaking, joint pain, and even hallucinations. This class of drugs is usually prescribed for premenstrual dysphoric disorder (PMDD) and major depression, rather than PMS. Sarafem, the first drug specifically marketed and approved as a PMDD treatment, is usually given daily for fourteen days before menstruation. However, a 2003 study showed that as soon as a woman stops taking this medication, symptoms returned the following month.

Antianxiety Drugs

Antianxiety drugs like Xanax are sometimes prescribed for women who don't get relief from their symptoms with SSRIs or other treatments. Antianxiety drugs work by depressing the central nervous system. Standard anti-anxiety drugs include benzodiazepines, such as alprazolam (Xanax) and buspirone (BuSpar). Benzodiazepines are addictive and have significant side effects such as drowsiness and a hung-over feeling. Buspirone is milder: it is not addictive and has fewer side effects, and evidence suggests it reduces PMS-induced irritability.

Should I See a Counselor?

If you're having trouble coping with PMS, one option is psychological counseling. The emotional aspects of PMS can be very troubling, and if stress, anger, or family issues are factors in your life, they probably just compound the problem.

As Chapter 1 illustrates, society expects women to become overly emotional during their premenstrual phase; and for some women, this two-week window may be the time they feel most able to vent. Counseling can provide a more workable framework for those emotions and can help women discover why they are angry, irritable, sad, and depressed. It can also teach women how to anticipate and cope with symptoms, how to communicate more effectively, and how to reduce stress.

There are several ways to find a counselor:

- **Ask your physician.** Your family physician or obstetrician-gynecologist may be able to refer you to a counselor who works with PMS patients.

- **Check your local hospital.** Some hospitals have PMS clinics, in which physicians and nurses treat the patient, provide nutrition and lifestyle information, and provide referrals to other professionals.
- **Check your college health clinic.** Many colleges and universities offer their students access to counseling and health information. If you're a college student, contact your school's health clinic. If you're not a student, you can still call to get referrals and information.
- **Call your local university.** Universities and colleges with psychology departments can be a great resource. The staff and faculty can point you in the right direction when you're looking for a PMS specialist.
- **Check online.** Many organizations offer a database of counselors who practice in your local area. For example, the publication *Psychology Today*, in partnership with *U.S. News & World Report*, a magazine known for its annual physician and hospital ranking, lists therapists and counselors in a number of cities.
- **Contact professional or certification organizations.** Psychologists and counselors are certified by the American Board of Professional Psychology. The ABPP Web site offers a directory of specialists.

CHAPTER 10

Risk Factors

BRAIN CHEMISTRY AND BIOLOGY aren't the only factors that determine whether you suffer from PMS, so do lifestyle choices, diet, and even the pace of modern life. In fact, the first course of treatment prescribed by doctors for premenstrual syndrome is to modify your lifestyle. Consider the role of your lifestyle in PMS, and what you might want to change. This chapter will discuss the choices you make in daily life that can actually lead to increased PMS symptoms.

Are You Making Yourself Sick?

Some women will find it difficult to imagine (and perhaps even more difficult to admit) that they might be making themselves feel worse. But PMS is exacerbated by all sorts of things—what and how we eat, whether we drink alcohol, our jobs, our relationships, our coping strategies, whether we exercise, and even society's expectations of us. No single factor causes PMS (after all, brain chemistry and biology are the primary drivers), but habits and choices nevertheless impact overall well-being and influence the degree to which women feel disabled by PMS.

The typical woman's lifestyle today is more stressful, harried, and unhealthy than ever. Thanks to technology like cell phones, PDAs, and laptop computers, women can work anywhere and anytime. The downside, of course, is that for many working women, there is no time off from the job. Society also expects women to be super-moms or super-working-moms. Of course, stress levels are sky high!

Add to this the availability and convenience of unhealthful foods, cramped schedules that leave little—if any—time for exercise, and the picture becomes clearer: women are becoming more overweight and less healthy than ever. This leaves most women more susceptible to PMS, and it can exacerbate the symptoms.

Stress

Stress, a well-known factor in PMS, is a widely studied aspect of modern life. It's everywhere: at work, at home caused by families, and even in social relationships. While some stress is necessary and even beneficial, too much unleashes a host of negative consequences on the body and the psyche.

There are three types of stress: psychological, physiological, and environmental:

Psychological stress
- Emotional or mental problems
- Trauma

Physiological stress
- Fatigue
- Injury
- Surgery
- Starvation
- Illness

Environmental stress
- Excessive sound
- Excessive light
- Heat
- Cold

Alert

Stress can depress the immune system and may be harmful to certain parts of the brain. Stress also affects multiple organ systems in the body, including the cardiovascular and glandular systems. Stress also makes women more vulnerable to PMS.

Good Stress

Though it seems unlikely at first glance, some stress is actually good for you. It challenges your body and your development as an individual. Stressing your muscles makes them grow, while stress in your personal life, such as deadlines and expectations, can motivate you to work harder and push your boundaries. Some stress may also be beneficial to health. In 2000, researchers at Ohio State University showed that short bursts of stress can actually enhance immune system response.

The sympathetic nervous system responds to threatening stimuli by preparing for danger (both real and imagined). Breathing, heart rate, and blood pressure increase, senses and memory become sharper, there is less sensitivity to pain, and the muscles and brain are fueled with oxygen-rich blood. When the stress is perceived as positive, it makes a person more alert, feeling challenged, focused, "juiced," or "in the zone."

Bad Stress

Chronic and excessive stress are entirely different matters. Stress is the body's response to danger, and if you feel constantly threatened, you deplete your mental and physical resources always trying to stay on alert. Too much stress makes you feel overwhelmed or powerless. Usually, the initial signs of this kind of negative stress are physical: you feel anxious or irritable, your head and muscles ache, you're preoccupied, and you may come down with a virus more easily. Of course, your PMS symptoms also usually worsen.

The following hormones and neurotransmitters are involved in the stress response:

- **Corticotropin-releasing hormone (CRH)** is released by the hypothalamus in response to a threatening stimulus. CRH triggers the release of cortisol.
- **Cortisol**, the primary stress hormone, cues various systems throughout the body, including the heart, lungs, and metabolism, to respond to a threat. The brain also releases the neurotransmitters dopamine, norepinephrine, and epinephrine.
- **Dopamine, norepinephrine and epinephrine (or adrenaline)** activate an area in the brain called the amgydala, which triggers an emotional response, such as fear, to the stressful stimulus. These chemical messengers also allow a person to react quickly by suppressing short-term memory, inhibition, rational thought, and the ability to handle complex social and intellectual tasks.

The Health Effects of Stress

Stress also contributes to serious illnesses and health conditions. For example, there is a growing body of evidence that stress contributes to heart disease. A British study of ten thousand civil servants found a link between chronic work stress and the symptoms of metabolic syndrome, a collection of health risk factors such as obesity and high blood pressure that can lead to heart disease, stroke, and diabetes.

Stress also contributes to asthma and bronchitis, can lead to gastrointestinal problems (such as ulcers and chronic diarrhea), is associated with high blood pressure, and can alter heart rhythms.

Many women with asthma often find their symptoms worsen in the premenstrual phase. A 1998 Danish study suggests that stress is partly to blame. Researchers examined the psychological and physical status of ten women with asthma during a six-month period and found that lowered resistance to stress and lowered resistance to infection combined to make bronchial activity worse.

 Fact

> There is evidence that many people with depression have high activity of the stress hormone CRH. Excess production of cortisol, the body's main stress hormone, leads to a rare disease called Cushing's syndrome.

In women, stress poses serious physical and mental problems. Chronic stress in women may reduce estrogen levels, which puts their cardiac health at risk. Many conditions that affect women disproportionately, such as eating disorders, irritable bowel syndrome, and depression, are linked to stress. Stress also has multiple effects on sexuality and reproduction. Stress can reduce libido and the ability to achieve orgasm; severely elevated cortisol levels can stop a woman's menstrual periods; and stress during pregnancy has been linked to a higher risk of miscarriage, especially early in the first trimester.

Social Stress

Relationships with others—family members, spouses, neighbors, coworkers, friends, or strangers—are a major source of stress. Any social situation can produce problems for some individuals, and certain groups of people are particularly vulnerable to social stress (e.g., children who are bullied; chronically ill adults without a support system; older adults who care for disabled children, spouses, or parents; and seniors whose spouses have died).

Top Stressors

In 1967, psychiatrist Thomas Holmes and Richard Rahe, a Navy scientist, created a scale of the most stressful events in a person's life, known as the Holmes-Rahe scale. For adults, the death of a spouse is the most stressful event, given a score of 100 points. Here is how some other events compare:

Stressful Events

Stressor	Point Value
Divorce	60 points
Menopause	60 points
Jail term or probation	60 points
Being fired	45 points
Working more than 40 hours per week	35 points
Foreclosure of a mortgage or loan	25 points
PMS	15 points
Winter holiday season	10 points

It's interesting that menopause is as stressful as a jail term and that, while it's at the low end of the scale, PMS merits its own entry!

Social stress can manifest itself as shyness, loneliness, intimidation, competitiveness, and hostility toward others. It affects both physical and mental health. People without support systems suffer more severe depression symptoms.

Reacting to Stress

It's simply not possible to avoid stress, nor is it even necessarily good. But it is possible to manage reactions to stress. Stress management is critical for women with severe PMS, since the more stressed they are, the worse their symptoms get (the corollary is that a woman who is prone to stress easily is also more likely to get PMS). Having a supportive partner and a strong social network are very important to managing both stress and PMS.

Men and women manage stress differently. While men favor a fight-or-flight approach, women would rather "tend and befriend," according to a 2000 study by researchers at the University of California, Los Angeles. Shelley Taylor, Ph.D., a psychology professor at UCLA, and her colleagues, reviewed dozens of studies of stress on animals and humans. They found that stressed females spent more time tending to vulnerable offspring than males did and theorized that endorphins and oxytocin, a female reproductive hormone, may play an important role in establishing this behavior. Women also befriend other women in times of stress.

When you are besieged by violent mood swings, feel anxious and depressed, when your body and head ache, and you feel physically uncomfortable or even ill, it helps tremendously to know there is someone who understands that your experience and feelings are genuine, even if they can't really do anything about it other than support you. In cases where social support is not enough of a boost, then therapy or counseling, which can help you find strategies to cope with stress, is appropriate.

Poor Diet

Like stress, a poor diet is not only connected to PMS, it is a pervasive social problem with serious health consequences. Each week, it seems, brings a news report or an article about how bad the typical high-fat, high-sugar, high-calorie American diet of fast food, soda, processed foods, and enormous portion sizes is. This diet has been blamed for an increase in chronic disease, including diabetes (especially type 2 diabetes), heart disease, and high blood pressure. Of course, obesity carries its own risks, such as gallbladder disease, depression, certain types of cancer, arthritis, sleep apnea, irregular menstrual cycles, pregnancy complications, and infertility.

 Alert

According to the U.S. surgeon general, a gain of eleven to eighteen pounds doubles a person's chance of developing type 2 diabetes compared to a person who has not gained weight.

The Danger in Comfort Foods

Turning to junk food—whether it's ice cream, pasta, chips, tubs of buttery popcorn, or mashed potatoes and gravy—is a time-honored tradition to ward off stress and depression and to self-manage those irritating PMS symptoms. Research shows these types of foods can reduce the effects of stress on the brain in the short-term.

When you eat these comfort foods, the sugar content (and remember, carbohydrates are metabolized as sugar) provides immediate energy and a big dose of pleasure (as serotonin floods the brain). This spike in blood sugar is followed by a quick drop that can lead to headache, dizziness, anxiety, and irritability. This roller-coaster ride in your bloodstream has long-term consequences: over time, a steady dose of this "comfort" therapy can lead to stress, exhaustion, and depression, as well as obesity.

 Alert

Obesity is strongly associated with PMS. A study of 874 women by researchers at Virginia Commonwealth University found that obese women, defined as having a body mass index of thirty or more, had three times the risk of PMS than nonobese women.

Unhealthy Lifestyle

Adopting a healthier lifestyle is one of the simplest and most effective things you can do to minimize the symptoms of PMS. Virtually every health and PMS expert says you should exercise regularly; eat more fruit, vegetables, and fiber; avoid caffeine, salt, sugar, and high-fat foods; and make time to relax. Yet this simple and direct advice is hard to follow, in part because it is so all-encompassing. It seems as though you need to change everything in your life to feel better. Wouldn't it be simpler just to take a pill?

Well, no. Both prescription and over-the-counter drugs treat the symptoms, not necessarily the cause of PMS. In addition, they can have side effects and may be costly to take over time. In contrast, a better diet, regular exercise, and learning to relax are inexpensive, have multiple benefits beyond PMS relief, and can prevent, rather than medicate, your symptoms. For many women, however, getting to a healthier lifestyle is an exercise in frustration that includes fad diets, unrealistic expectations, and a lack of information

Fad Diets

Dieting is an American hobby, and fad diets are a particular favorite because they promise quick and dramatic results. Although it may be tempting to succumb to the latest diet craze, it can lead to weight cycling, also known as yo-yo dieting. That's because diets that promise quick results tend to overemphasize a particular food and keep portions unrealistically small, so that you quickly feel deprived—and when you feel deprived, you're more likely to cheat.

 Fact

Americans are eating more—a lot more—than they used to eat. According to the U.S. Department of Agriculture, Americans consumed an average of 300 calories more in 2000 than they did in 1985. That's a 12 percent increase in 15 years. Refined grains, such as those found in processed foods, accounted for 46 percent of that increase!

Weight cycling can also have negative effects on PMS. First, fad or excessive diets are nutritionally bad because by limiting certain types of foods, they also exclude the nutrients associated with those foods. They may also pose serious health risks. For example, high-protein diets tend to have a high fat content, which may harm the cardiovascular system.

Second, the weight lost on a fad diet is usually caused by dehydration (especially if you drop several pounds in a week). While that may be good news if you get bloated during PMS, dehydration means you lose electrolytes, the salts and minerals that control the fluid levels in your body. An electrolyte imbalance reduces your circulating blood volume, which means your heart has to beat harder to pump blood to your organs, and your body is less able to control blood pressure. Third, the stress of losing and then regaining weight is significant, and increased stress means more severe PMS.

Family History: Why It Matters

Your family and personal medical history offer important clues in diagnosing and managing PMS. They can tell you if you're likely to suffer more intense PMS symptoms or if you're at risk for other illnesses that worsen or mimic PMS, such as depression or irritable bowel syndrome.

Essential

A 1987 study showed that doctors considered medical history to be the most important diagnostic tool, better even than diagnostic technology. Although new technologies have since been developed, many doctors still feel the same way. A new effort by the U.S. surgeon general, for example, urges people to complete their family history.

These histories also provide clues such as whether you should be screened for certain health conditions, how you might react to certain medications, and if you're at risk for potential drug interactions. In addition, your family and personal health histories typically include information on your environment and your habits. Together, this information paints a portrait for your doctor that can be used to establish a course of action.

Your PMS health history should include the following:

- A record of your PMS symptoms

- A history of any PMS-like symptoms (even if they didn't occur during the premenstrual phase)
- Your menstrual history, including the date you started menstruating, the length of your cycle, and any problems associated with your periods
- Your pregnancy history
- Your sexual history (e.g., any sexually transmitted diseases)
- Any family members with PMS
- A mental health history (depression, anxiety, etc.)
- Any chronic conditions
- Drugs you are taking
- Supplements you are taking
- Your habits: whether you smoke, exercise, drink alcohol, and information on your diet

 Fact

According to the U.S. surgeon general, although 96 percent of people believe that knowing their health history is important, only one-third have actually gathered it and written it down.

Minimizing Risk Factors

Lose weight if you have to. Cut back on alcohol and work aerobic activity into your daily or weekly schedule. But how should you go about all these lifestyle-changing activities, exactly?

Start Slowly

Weight-loss experts and physicians recommend a balanced diet, with nutritionally sound choices. For many women, this sounds boring and impossible. The recommendations don't usually include favorites like pasta, brownies, or cheese pizza, and overhauling your entire diet is overwhelming.

Instead of resigning yourself to a boring diet, or trying to change everything you eat, start small. Target one item in your diet and replace it with a better choice; then move on to the next. For example, cut out white bread and replace it with whole wheat, or switch your soft drink to a bottle of water and see how that works for a few weeks. You may be surprised to find that, having made only those two minor changes, you will feel more full (and therefore eat less), consume much less sugar, and have more energy. Then go from there.

The same goes for exercise. Don't attempt to do everything at once, but do try something: yoga, Pilates, walking, dancing, swimming, jogging, racquetball. Even once a week is a start, especially if you are sedentary all day. Take a power walk during your lunch break or walk the stairs in your building for ten minutes.

Become Informed

Read, ask, listen, and learn. Talk to your doctor and your friends with PMS. Find articles and books on your symptoms. Be your own health advocate. Chart your menstrual cycles and your PMS symptoms. Becoming informed will help you make the best decisions on how to treat your PMS symptoms. Should you go to a medical doctor or a counselor? Do you want to try prescription drugs, or do you prefer alternative remedies? Only you can provide the best answer to these questions.

CHAPTER 11

Premenstrual Dysphoric Disorder

UNLESS YOU'RE LIVING WITH IT, you probably don't know what premenstrual dysphoric disorder is. Most women don't. But there are millions of women for whom the one or two weeks before their periods are an absolute nightmare: crying fits, crushing depression, anxiety, and physical pain so severe it disrupts their lives. But there is help. This chapter will discuss the signs and symptoms of PMDD, how it differs from PMS, and what kinds of treatments are available.

PMDD Is Not PMS

Premenstrual dysphoric disorder (PMDD) is not normal PMS. It is PMS on steroids, a severe and debilitating disorder that is similar to depression. Health professionals define PMDD as a mood disorder that affects women in the luteal phase of their menstrual cycle. But what does this mean?

First, PMDD-related symptoms, like regular PMS, are cyclical. They start seven to fourteen days before your period is due and stop once you get your period. Second, PMDD sufferers primarily experience mood symptoms such as depression, anxiety, mood swings, or irritability. That's not to say that they don't experience other PMS symptoms like bloating or food cravings, they do. But no matter how severe the physical symptoms, a diagnosis of PMDD requires at least one mood symptom that is not related to another disorder. In other words, women who have mood symptoms such as depression throughout their entire cycle do not have PMDD, even if their symptoms worsen in the premenstrual phase. Instead, they may have another mood disorder entirely. True PMDD symptoms cease after a woman gets her period.

Finally, *not* every woman who feels depressed or suffers from mood swings or anxiety before her period has PMDD. It's a matter of severity. Although PMS interferes with your life, it is manageable. PMS and PMDD both interfere with a woman's ability to deal with day-to-day life, such as maintaining personal relationships or going to work, but there is a very specific set of criteria for PMDD and the symptoms are much more severe. (Chapter 12 outlines the diagnostic criteria for PMDD)

Many women, even those with severe symptoms, aren't aware of PMDD. A 2000 survey of 500 women, commissioned by the Society for Women's Health Research, a nonprofit advocacy group, produced the following results:

- 84 percent did not know severe PMS symptoms have officially been recognized as PMDD and that such symptoms can be diagnosed and treated
- 45 percent never discussed PMS with their doctors
- 24 percent who described their symptoms as strong or severe were among those who were unaware of PMDD
- 24 percent who described their symptoms as strong or severe felt their doctors would not take their complaints seriously

What Is PMDD?

The Diagnostic and Statistical Manual of Mental Disorders, used by health professionals to diagnose mental disorders, first listed PMDD in 1994, defining it as a "depressive disorder not otherwise specified." However, PMDD is included in the manual's appendix, which means that it is not an official diagnosis, only that it has a common definition. There is ongoing research on PMDD, and experts hope eventually to have the disorder listed as a separate diagnostic category.

Before making a diagnosis, your doctor will ask you to chart your symptoms over at least two cycles (Chapter 13 explains how to chart your symptoms). According to the American Psychiatric Association, to be diagnosed with PMDD, you must have five or more of the following symptoms during the week before your period; the symptoms start to diminish shortly after you get your period; and they disappear completely in the week after your period. This is the critical differentiator between PMDD and other mood disorders: the symptoms disappear—not just lessen in intensity—after you get your period. These symptoms include:

- Markedly depressed mood, feelings of hopelessness, or negative thoughts
- Marked anxiety, tension, a feeling of being on edge
- Marked mood swings (suddenly feeling sad, weepy, or being sensitive to rejection)
- Persistent and marked anger and irritability, or increased personal conflicts
- Decreased interest in usual activities, such as work, school, friends, or hobbies
- Feeling that you have problems concentrating
- Feeling lethargic, easily fatigued, or having a marked lack of energy
- Having sleep problems (insomnia or excessive sleepiness)
- Feeling overwhelmed or out-of-control
- Physical symptoms such as breast tenderness, bloating, headache, joint and muscle pain

These mood and physical symptoms must interfere with work, school, or your usual activities. For example, they must be significant enough that you miss work or are less productive, or avoid school or activities. In addition, these mood and physical symptoms can't be attributed to another disorder, such as depression or panic disorder, which may become worse during the premenstrual phase.

Who Gets PMDD?

Only about 3 to 8 percent of women who report PMS-like symptoms have PMDD; nevertheless, that's still anywhere from 3 to 5 million women or up to one in twenty women with regular menstrual periods.

PMDD has a biological basis, but it is also affected by psychological, social, and cultural factors, such as being aware of premenstrual syndrome, stress, and socioeconomic status.

If you have a history of depression or postpartum depression, you are more likely to suffer from PMDD. Between 30 and 76 percent of women diagnosed with PMDD have a lifetime history of depression, compared to 15 percent of women of similar age without PMDD. Women with a personal or family history of mood disorders are also at higher risk of developing PMDD.

Other risk factors for PMDD include:

- Experiencing traumatic events, such as rape
- Other existing anxiety disorders, such as seasonal affective disorder
- Premenstrual mood changes
- History of sexual abuse
- Past or present domestic violence

While there is no definitive explanation for PMDD, the most common theory is that PMDD is an abnormal reaction to normal hormonal fluctuations in the central nervous system. The abnormal reaction affects brain chemistry, especially serotonin. For example, research shows that women with PMDD have reduced serotogenic activity. The cyclical nature of PMDD also suggests that the sex hormones estrogen and progesterone alter the levels of neurotransmitters, including serotonin. In addition, the success of selective serotonin reuptake inhibitors (SSRIs) such as Sarafem or Sertraline in treating PMDD symptoms makes a strong case for the importance of serotonin in PMDD.

Finally, there is some evidence there may be a genetic component to PMDD and PMS. Women whose mothers had PMS are nearly twice as likely to have PMS themselves—70 percent compared to 37 percent of women with PMS whose mothers did not have PMS. Identical twins are more than twice as likely to have PMDD than fraternal twins; 93 percent of identical twins share PMDD, while only 44 percent of fraternal twins do.

Theories on the Causes of PMDD

There are several major theories used to explain the causes of PMDD:

- **Ovarian hormone theory:** PMDD is caused by an imbalance in the ratio of estrogen to progesterone, especially a relative deficiency in progesterone. Studies on this theory have been inconclusive.
- **Serotonin theory:** Normal hormonal fluctuations cause changes in a woman's brain chemistry, particularly in the serotonin system, causing PMDD symptoms. This is currently the leading theory.
- **Psychosocial theory:** PMS and PMDD are conscious manifestations of a woman's unconscious conflicts about her role in society.
- **Cognitive–social learning theory:** Many women are psychologically averse to their periods and have negative or extreme thoughts that reinforce their aversion to premenstrual symptoms. In response, they develop inappropriate coping strategies, such as mood swings or overeating, which reduce their stress temporarily but also set them up to repeat the process month after month.

Signs and Symptoms

Typically, women with PMDD have severe mood and physical symptoms in the week before their period. These symptoms include sadness and crying; nervousness, anxiety or irritability; mood swings, and problems concentrating and paying attention. They can also feel overwhelmed, have strong food cravings, sleep problems, fatigue, joint and muscle pain, bloating, and headaches. Typically, irritability is the most prominent and disabling symptom.

 ## Fact

PMDD symptoms are burdensome and disrupt women's relationships. A survey of 1,022 women, published in the *Journal of Women's Health & Gender-Based Research*, found that 92 percent of women with PMDD reported social interference, especially in their relationships with their husbands and children compared to women with PMS.

As in PMS, in PMDD the symptoms are tied to your menstrual cycle, so they disappear when your period begins. However, in PMDD, you experience more symptoms and the symptoms are more severe than in PMS (severe enough to interfere with work, school, or interpersonal relationships), and you must have them over at least two consecutive months. Women who have PMDD, rather than an underlying mood disorder, do not experience any physical or mental symptoms for seven to ten days after their menstrual cycle every month.

PMDD's Different Patterns

There is more than one pattern to PMDD: symptoms can last for one week or two, they can appear full-force and then disappear, or they can start gradually and worsen over time. Common patterns include symptoms that begin at ovulation and worsen gradually until you get your period; symptoms that begin at ovulation and persist throughout your entire period (that is, they don't end just before or immediately after your period); and symptoms that appear briefly at ovulation, clear up, and then reappear in the week before your period. A diagnosis of PMDD, assuming that it meets all the other criteria for symptoms (outlined in Chapter 12), requires that symptoms occur in the week before your period.

It May Not Be PMDD

However, sometimes what appears to be PMDD is something else entirely. As many as 40 percent of women who seek treatment for PMDD do not actually have the disorder. Instead, they may have a medical or psychiatric condition that comes and goes, or a psychiatric condition that gets worse during the premenstrual phase, rather than a separate case of PMDD.

 Alert

Women overwhelmingly underdiagnose their PMDD! The study that found women with PMDD have more social interference than women with PMS also found that, compared to using *DSM-IV* criteria, women were much less likely to self-diagnose as having severe premenstrual symptoms. Only 4.9 percent of 1,022 women self-reported severe symptoms, but a *DSM-IV*-adapted approach identified 11.3 percent of the same group as actually having PMDD.

There are a number of medical and psychiatric conditions that can be confused with PMDD, including major depression, minor depression (also known as dysthemia), generalized anxiety disorder, social anxiety disorder, bipolar disorder, anemia, chronic fatigue syndrome, hypothyroidism, diabetes, seizure disorders, autoimmune disorders, perimenopausal mood symptoms, allergy, collagen vascular disease, and endometriosis. That's why proper diagnosis is so important.

Diagnosing PMDD

In some ways, PMDD is a diagnosis of exclusion. There's no laboratory test for PMDD, so doctors typically consider a patient's medical history, a PMS diary, and self-reported symptoms. They use laboratory tests such as thyroid function tests, follicle-stimulating hormone levels, and complete blood cell counts to exclude other possible health conditions (such as anemia, thyroid disorders, or perimenopause) before diagnosing PMDD.

Differences Between PMS and PMDD

PMS and PMDD differ in degree. Not only are mood symptoms more severe, researchers have found further differences between PMDD sufferers and other women, both with and without PMS.

For one, women with PMDD have greater pain sensitivity than women with PMS. In a 2000 study of fifty-four women, twenty-seven with PMS and twenty-seven with PMDD, psychiatric experts at the University of North Carolina found that women with PMDD had a lower pain threshold than women with PMS when their blood flow to their arms was restricted using blood pressure cuffs. PMDD sufferers also had shorter times of pain tolerance than the women with PMS. One reason may be that the PMDD sufferers had low levels of beta-endorphins in their blood. These endorphins are natural painkillers, and PMDD sufferers had levels that were 30 percent lower than women with PMS.

 Fact

PMDD, which tends to develop in women in their late twenties, can affect between 1,400 and 2,800 days in a woman's lifetime, or four to eight years' worth of symptomatic days.

Women with PMDD are also much likelier to have been sexually abused than other women. Between 50 and 60 percent of women with PMDD have histories of physical or sexual abuse, while experts estimate the rates for the general population are much lower at 20 to 25 percent. PMDD sufferers may also have dysregulated stress response systems. A 1998 study at the University of North Carolina tested the stress responses of twelve women with PMDD and twelve healthy women and found that women with PMDD had chronic stress in their daily lives. Blood tests showed abnormally elevated levels of the stress hormone norepinephrine and abnormally low levels of cortisol. The high levels of norepinephrine remained constant, regardless of the day of the women's cycles.

Mood Disorders

Distinguishing between PMDD and other mood disorders can be very difficult. The symptoms of major depressive disorder (MDD), bipolar disorder, and dysthemia often worsen during a woman's luteal phase, which gives the appearance that the conditions are tied to the menstrual cycle even when they aren't. PMDD is also sometimes confused with panic disorder and generalized anxiety disorder. (Chapter 8 describes these disorders in more detail.)

 Question

Why is it so critical to distinguish between a mood disorder and PMDD, especially if the mood symptoms are similar?
Accurate diagnosis of mental disorders is critical for appropriate treatment. PMDD is treated differently than major depression, with which it is often confused. For example, PMDD can be treated using intermittent doses of the SSRI fluoxetine; the drug may be given only during the luteal phase. In contrast, major depression is typically treated with continuous (daily) dosing of SSRIs (both fluoxetine and other types of SSRIs), frequently in conjunction with therapy.

PMDD Treatments

Most physicians will recommend that women first modify their life-style, such as changing their diet and increasing exercise, before they prescribe drugs for PMDD. For women who need more help than life-style changes offer, however, there are plenty of treatment options

Nondrug Treatments

In general, nondrug treatments can improve the patient's coping strategies or affect brain chemistry. For example, light therapy seems to increase serotonin activity, which is implicated in depression and PMDD. Some nondrug treatments for PMDD include:

- **Relaxation therapy:** Some research shows relaxation techniques, which help decrease heart rate, blood pressure, and slow breathing, are helpful in reducing the physical symptoms of PMDD.
- **Light therapy:** At least one study has demonstrated that thirty minutes of bright light reduces emotional and physical premenstrual symptoms.
- **Cognitive-behavioral treatment:** This treatment teaches patients to recognize, examine, and replace negative thought patterns with positive ones and can help reduce PMDD-related anger and negative emotions. Some research supports the positive effects of cognitive therapy on PMS symptoms.
- **Sleep deprivation:** Total sleep deprivation for one night is a therapy used to treat depression, providing short-term help to as many as 50 percent of depressed patients. Researchers don't know why manipulating the sleep cycle improves mood, but it may have to do with disturbances in the dream sleep cycle, which are common in depressed patients. Research now suggests this type of treatment may be just as effective for PMDD patients. Sleep deprivation therapy only provides short-term benefits, but studies now suggest the resultant mood improvements can be maintained by daily light therapy or certain drugs.

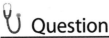 Question

What is sleep deprivation therapy?
Sleep deprivation is used to treat patients with depressive disorder at the beginning of their depressive episodes. Patients are kept awake all night and stay awake until the following night. This strategy improves mood in 50 to 80 percent of patients and may prevent the depressive episode from fully developing. However, up to 90 percent of people relapse immediately after the next period of sleep.

Vitamins, Supplements, and Diet

Diet changes and dietary supplements have been shown to improve many physical and some mood symptoms in PMDD and PMS patients. Vitamin B6, magnesium, calcium, and evening primrose oil have been studied as possible PMS and PMDD treatments. While data supporting vitamin B6 is limited and of poor quality, small doses may be helpful in reducing symptoms. Calcium supplements in the luteal phase of the premenstrual cycle can reduce bloating and pain, improve mood, and reduce food cravings; and a daily 200-milligram dose of magnesium has been shown to reduce bloating. Evening primrose oil is often recommended by alternative medical practitioners and is popular in Europe and Australia to treat breast tenderness; however, clinical studies have not shown it to be an effective PMS remedy.

Diet and dietary supplements are also thought to be helpful in improving some of the symptoms of PMDD. One recent nonrandomized trial found that a low-fat vegetarian diet reduced PMS symptoms, but there is insufficient data on dietary supplements to recommend them as a treatment.

Hormones

Hormone treatments include progesterone, birth control pills, and drugs used to suppress the ovarian cycle. The theory is that women can't experience PMDD if they're not ovulating. Some common hormone treatments include:

- **Progesterone:** A number of studies have found that progesterone is no better than a placebo in treating PMS, while data on synthetic progesterone-like drugs, such as dydrogesterone, are conflicting.
- **GnRH analogues:** Drugs such as Lupron and Synarel manipulate ovulation by shutting down the ovaries. They are commonly used in infertility treatments and more recently to save the eggs of women undergoing chemotherapy. Clinical trials have shown they have a beneficial effect on PMS symptoms, but because there is a high risk of osteoporosis if they are used for more than six months, GnRH analogues aren't appropriate as a long-term therapy.
- **Danazol:** Used to suppress the ovarian cycle, this drug reduces premenstrual symptoms, but it has its own set of adverse effects, including weight gain, hot flashes, mood instability, vaginal dryness, and an intensification of masculine characteristics, which limit its use as a PMDD drug.
- **Birth control pills:** Oral contraceptives seem to alleviate the physical symptoms of PMDD, such as breast tenderness and bloating, but do not affect psychological symptoms.

In some women, the side effects of oral contraceptives worsen or mimic PMDD symptoms. In 2006, the FDA approved a new oral contraceptive that may have some significant benefits for PMDD. The birth control pill, called YAZ, has more days of active hormones than other low-dose contraceptives, which means that women experience fewer hormone fluctuations and fewer symptoms. With typical low-dose oral contraceptives, women take hormones for twenty-one days and then a placebo pill for seven days. In contrast, women on YAZ go off hormones for four days only. In a clinical study, 450 women with PMDD took either YAZ or a placebo pill. The results were significant: 48 percent of the women taking YAZ reported significant improvement in their PMDD symptoms, compared with 36 percent of women taking a placebo pill. However, YAZ contains a progestin called drospirenone, which may increase potassium levels and can lead to serious problems for women with kidney, liver, or adrenal disease.

 Fact

Don't get confused. YAZ and Yasmin are two different brands of oral contraceptives that sound alike and combine the same hormones, ethinyl estradiol (an estrogen) and drospirenone (a progestin). However, YAZ has twenty-four days of active hormones and contains a 20-mcg dose of the ethinyl estradiol, while Yasmin has the standard twenty-one days of active hormones and contains 30 mcgs of ethinyl estradiol.

Diuretics and NSAIDs

Diuretics and nonsteroidal anti-inflammatory drugs come in both prescription and over-the-counter versions. NSAIDs are helpful in reducing inflammation, while diuretics, such as spironolactone, reduce swelling, bloating, and weight gain.

SSRIs

Selective serotogenic reuptake inhibitors are becoming the drug of choice for PMDD. Several research trials have shown that SSRIs are both effective and have minimal side effects. A common SSRI is fluoxetine (sold under the brand name Sarafem or Prozac). Fluoxetine has been shown to reduce tension, irritability, and depression but is not as effective on physical symptoms. Its most common side effect is sexual dysfunction, such as decreased libido and the inability to orgasm. Sertaline, another SSRI, reduces both behavioral and physical symptoms, according to two randomized controlled trials. Paroxetine-controlled release has also proven effective when given during the luteal phase.

L. Essential

Some other drugs including dual-action antidepressants such as nefazodone, non-SSRI antidepressants such as bupropion and clomipramine, and anxiolytics (anti-anxiety medications) such as buspirone have all been shown to reduce one or more symptoms of PMDD.

Surgical Options

Surgery is a treatment of last resort for PMDD because it ends a woman's fertility, and it cues the onset of menopause, which has its own set of physical symptoms. However, a hysterectomy (the surgical removal of the uterus), along with the removal of the ovaries (known as a bilateral oophorectomy) cures PMDD, while a hysterectomy alone can reduce symptoms.

CHAPTER 12

PMDD Self-Test

IF YOU SUSPECT YOU MIGHT HAVE PMDD, consult your doctor; but first, gather more information. How can you be sure your symptoms are not simply PMS or are caused by some other illness? What will you discuss with your doctor? Is there some sort of test you can take that tells you if you have PMDD? This chapter will explore the questions and criteria you need to know to confirm PMDD suspicions, as well as how to chart your symptoms.

Could It Be PMDD?

Suspecting that you may have PMDD is the first step in treating it, but distinguishing between PMDD and PMS, or between PMDD and some other illnesses, is not all that simple.

For one, with its wide array of physical and psychological symptoms, PMS itself can be disabling, making you achy, bloated, moody, and depressed. Many women think there isn't any point in treating PMS. If they just wait it out, they believe the symptoms will eventually go away.

PMDD is an under-recognized disorder. The majority of women with severe symptoms don't even know there is such a condition—let alone that they have it. In this context, it's easy to assume that your severe symptoms are just part of "normal" PMS. Feeling that you can't get out of bed or that you're mired in hopelessness is not normal PMS; it is PMDD.

While some women may understand the severity of their symptoms, it might not occur to them to link those symptoms to their menstrual cycle. Instead, they write off the emotional turmoil and physical symptoms they are experiencing as responses to stressful events in their lives. Or they are so immersed in their feelings that they simply cannot be objective about what might be causing their symptoms. This is where the objectivity of a partner or family member becomes valuable. The people in your life may be able to demonstrate to you what you can't see for yourself: that your symptoms aren't normal and that they are related to your period.

PMS Versus PMDD

PMDD is an extreme version of PMS, especially in terms of the mood symptoms. Charting the similarities and differences between regular PMS and PMDD might look something like this:

PMS	PMDD
Mild depression	Significant depression
Sadness	Hopelessness
Irritability	Rages
Anxiety	Crippling anxiety that interferes with social life, work, or relationships
Mood swings	Crying fits, feeling crazy

Women with PMDD describe all-night crying jags, going into rages (even to the point of throwing things), feeling as though they are going crazy or being shackled by such despair they don't even want to live. These are extreme feelings and in no way should they be discounted.

What Next?

Confusion about what symptoms constitute PMDD is just the first hurdle to getting treatment. The second is getting over a reluctance to speak to a doctor for fear that he or she may just dismiss your symptoms or getting past the assumption that you can handle things on your own.

According to a 2000 survey commissioned by the Society for Women's Health Research, 90 percent of the women who said they were reluctant to seek treatment even if they thought they had PMDD felt they could cope on their own, while about 25 percent of those women felt their doctors would not take their complaints seriously.

 Fact

When the Society for Women's Health Research surveyed 500 women in 2000, they found that women with PMDD are more likely to have symptoms month in and month out, compared with women who have PMS—26 percent of women with PMDD versus 5 percent of women with PMS.

Being at the mercy of your overwhelming feelings is not healthy, especially when these feelings interfere with your everyday life or when they are harmful to your relationships.

Diagnostic Criteria

So now that you suspect your severe depression, rages, and extreme mood swings are symptoms of PMDD, will your doctor agree with your assessment? Physicians look for very specific criteria before they diagnose PMDD, including having at least one mood symptom that is unrelated to another medical condition. Frequently, the symptoms of mood disorders worsen during the premenstrual phase and can be confused with PMDD. Your doctor will want to exclude this possibility. According to the *DSM-IV*, PMDD is diagnosed when a woman has at least five of the eleven following symptoms over the course of a year:

- Depression, hopelessness, possibly even suicidal thoughts
- Tension or anxiety
- Panic attacks
- Mood swings, marked by periods of crying
- Persistent anger or irritability that affects other people
- Difficulty concentrating
- Lack of interest in previously enjoyed activities
- Fatigue or low energy
- Increased appetite, food cravings, or binge eating
- Insomnia or hypersomnia (excessive sleepiness)
- Feeling overwhelmed or out-of-control

These symptoms are present most of the time in the last week of the luteal phase, start to fade or disappear when your period begins, and are absent in the week after your period. In addition, in order to be diagnosed with PMDD, these symptoms must disturb your social life, job, or relationships, and they must last for at least two consecutive months.

Charting

A premenstrual symptom chart is as close as you can get to a test of PMDD because it shows what your symptoms are, their severity, and when they occur. If you haven't done so already, your doctor will ask you to chart your symptoms before diagnosing you with PMDD.

In addition to charting your symptoms, your doctor may ask you to record your basal body temperature to confirm that your symptoms occur during the luteal phase. To do this, use a special thermometer (available in most pharmacies) to take your temperature the first thing in the morning, before you get out of bed. Charting is beneficial for a number of reasons: it will help you identify what symptoms you have and when they occur to confirm that they are indeed tied to your menstrual phase; it will allow you to plan for days that you know you will be stressed (which may make you feel more in control of your PMDD); and it can help rule out other illnesses that may be causing your symptoms. In other words, it is a tool that lays out in black and white the jumble of physical and emotional symptoms you experience on a recurring basis. With several months' worth of charts, you'll be able to spot any patterns that emerge.

L. Essential

Women who want to increase their chances of conceiving frequently monitor their ovulation by charting their basal body temperature. Typically, your basal or resting body temperature dips slightly before ovulation and then peaks once you have ovulated due to elevated progesterone.

Let's say that you feel depressed and irritable most months, but some months you also feel bloated and achy. If you rely on your memory of your symptoms, the information is likely less accurate. Perhaps you remember the symptoms as being more or less severe than they actually were, or maybe you think you felt bloated for the first few days and then started feeling irritable. Charting will help you discover the real pattern. It may turn out that your physical symptoms appear late in the game, while your mood symptoms are constant, never having quite gone away, only intensifying around your period. The diagnosis may not be PMDD at all, but dysthemia, irritable bowel syndrome, or something else.

How to Chart

Charting your symptoms is a simple process. All you need is a note-pad and a pen. If you know your menstrual cycle, you will be able to keep a combination menstrual diary and premenstrual symptom chart based on the number of days in your cycle. If you're not sure of the length of your cycle, you may have to keep a PMS chart that lists your symptoms and a separate menstrual cycle chart. Once you're sure of your regular menstrual pattern, you should be able to combine both charts. If you're not sure of your menstrual cycle, organize your PMS chart based on the days of the month (between twenty-eight and thirty-one days). In other words, track your PMS symptoms according to the calendar. In contrast, your menstrual chart would only have as many days as your menstrual cycle, whether that's twenty-one, twenty-nine, or thirty-two days. (See Chapter 13 for more information on how to keep a menstrual diary.)

Charts: A Step-by-Step Process

First, create separate entries for each day in your cycle. On average, this will be about twenty-eight days, but this number could vary dramatically—as short as twenty-one days or as long as thirty-five days (typically considered the top range of the normal menstrual cycle). If you're keeping the information on one sheet, list the days vertically, along the left side of the page: 1, 2, 3, 4, ... and so forth.

Next, list the mood symptoms used to diagnose PMDD across the top of the page: irritability/anger, depression, anxiety, tension, mood swings, panic attacks, feeling out of control. Then list the cognitive, emotional, and physical symptoms: difficulty concentrating, social withdrawal (a lack of interest in previously enjoyed activities), crying, fatigue, headaches, food cravings, achiness, breast tenderness, bloating/swelling, and cramps.

Following is an example:

Sample PMS Symptom Chart

Cycle Day	Irritability/ anger	Depression	Bloating	Headaches
1	0	0	0	0
2	0	0	0	0
3	0	0	0	0
4	0	0	0	0
5	0	0	0	0
6	0	0	0	0
7	0	0	0	0
8	1	0	0	0
9	0	1	0	0
10	0	0	0	1
11	1	0	1	0
12	1	1	0	0
13	2	1	0	0
14	2	2	3	2
15	1	2	2	0
16	2	1	0	1
17	2	2	1	1
18	1	2	1	0
19	1	1	2	2
20	3	2	2	1
21	2	2	2	2
22	1	1	2	3
23	3	2	2	2
24	3	3	2	2
25	3	4	3	2
26	3	3	3	2
27	4	3	3	3
28	4	4	3	2

Once you get your period, start a new chart, beginning again with day 1.

Adjust the chart to accommodate the actual number of days in your cycle and list all the potential symptoms. If you experience any new symptom, be sure to add them to your chart so you can track them as well, and consult your doctor. There are many conditions, allergies and asthma among them, that may worsen during your pre-menstrual phase.

This will allow you to draw a grid, with a space for each symptom on each day.

Next, assign yourself a severity scale, for example, 0 through 4, or 0 through 5. Use this scale to rate your symptoms: 0 indicates you don't have the symptom; 1 means you have the symptom, but it has a minimal effect; 2 means the symptom is moderate, but doesn't affect your routine; 3 indicates the symptom is bothersome enough to affect your routine; 4 means it is severe; and 5 means it is overwhelming.

You can also keep your symptom chart in a notebook rather than on a single piece of paper. In this case, you might use a separate page for each day and then simply write down your symptoms for that day and rate them according to severity. For example, page eighteen (for day eighteen) might read: crying 4, bloating 2, irritability 10!

When charting you have a choice: you can either use preprinted charts or homemade versions; both have their pros and cons. Pre-printed charts, whether provided by your doctor or one of the many downloadable versions on the Internet, are convenient and easy to use. However, they are not as customizable as a chart you make yourself. Preprinted charts can also be hard to read, especially if you have vision problems.

In contrast, a handwritten or handmade chart allows you a lot of flexibility. You can customize your symptoms and the severity scale and have lots of space for handwritten notes. However, make sure you are using the ratings consistently and in the same way. Write down the definitions of each rating to serve as a constant reference for yourself and to show your health-care providers exactly what you mean by those ratings.

Charting Medications and Treatments

Even if you've never talked to your doctor about your premenstrual symptoms, more than likely you've tried to cope with them somehow (e.g., by taking medications, avoiding certain foods, or even taking a warm bath). In some cases, these strategies helped, while in others they had no effect.

This information can be a valuable addition to your symptom chart. As you rate your symptoms, jot down if you've taken anything for them, whether it relieved your symptoms, and whether it had any side effects. This will help you and your doctor understand, if you are consistent in applying lifestyle changes, whether you might be suffering from any reactions to medications (i.e., if you take a lot of NSAIDs, such as ibuprofen, and your symptom chart reveals you frequently suffer from indigestion, then you might be experiencing a side effect of too many NSAIDs), if there is a potential for negative drug interactions, or even if you may be suffering from other health conditions.

Key Questions

As you discuss your symptoms with your health-care provider, questions may develop. For your initial meeting, however, here are some of the most common questions about PMDD and some preliminary answers.

I'm embarrassed to seek treatment for my premenstrual symptoms. Is this normal?

Unfortunately, yes. A great many women don't seek treatment because they are embarrassed about having a premenstrual illness or a mood disorder. Society tends to stigmatize people with mental illness, in part because of so many misconceptions about what causes it and also because people often assume that mental illness causes people to be violent. In addition, many people in our society remain squeamish about anything having to do with the menstrual cycle. However, don't let embarrassment stand in the way of getting help for your symptoms. PMDD is a real and treatable illness.

How does PMDD impact my family?

Mood symptoms, such as depression, which predominate in PMDD, have a pronounced effect on your relationships with others, including spouses and children. A woman in the grips of a mood disorder has trouble relating to and interacting with her spouse and her children. As a result, spouses tend to get angry while children and adolescents feel insecure and develop behavior problems.

I have very severe mood symptoms. Should I go see a psychiatrist or should I stick with my gynecologist?

That depends. If you have not yet spoken with your doctor, either your gynecologist or your primary care provider, about your PMDD, you might want to start there. He or she will be able to help you assess your symptoms and suggest a course of action that does not rely on drugs. He or she can also prescribe drugs if necessary. However, if you suspect you might have depression, bipolar illness, or another mood disorder, you might be better off with a psychiatrist. Psychiatrists are also more experienced in distinguishing and treating depressive disorder than your primary care physician or OB/GYN. Finally, a psychiatrist is likely to treat PMDD with different drugs than your OB-GYN would.

May I try alternative medicine to treat my PMDD or do I have to take SSRIs?

Any time you have significant mood symptoms, you should see your physician for assessment and possible treatment. However, if you are strongly opposed to standard medicine and are comfortable using herbal products (which are not subject to FDA oversight and scrutiny), you may want to try taking chasteberry.

A 2001 German study of 178 women found that a 20-milligram tablet daily of Agnus castus, the active fruit extract in chasteberry, helped alleviate premenstrual symptoms better than a placebo. The women in the study received daily either a 20-milligram tablet or a placebo. Researchers found that 52 percent of the women receiving Agnus castus reported improvement, compared with 24 percent of the placebo group. This result is similar to that of improvements reported for SSRIs.

What are the side effects of SSRIs?

The side effects of these medications include nervousness, insomnia, sexual dysfunction, restlessness, nausea, and diarrhea. For this reason, most doctors prescribe a low dose at first and then increase it slowly as needed. This is also why it's important to change medications gradually if necessary. If you experience significant side effects from your medication, don't discontinue it without your doctor's supervision.

What if I do nothing? Does PMDD end on its own?

If you wait long enough, menopause will eventually put an end to your PMDD symptoms. But depending on your age, you may be waiting a long, long time. Finally, your PMDD may actually be a different mood disorder or may be complicated by another mood disorder. In this case, your symptoms will not spontaneously end at menopause but will continue to affect your life.

What to Expect at the Doctor's Office

Most medical professionals prefer to treat PMDD with less intensive or invasive treatments before moving on to more powerful drugs, which typically have unpleasant side effects. This means getting relief from PMDD can be a long process that involves several approaches. You can save yourself some time by charting your symptoms before seeing your doctor.

Here's a rundown of how your doctor will assess and treat your severe premenstrual symptoms:

1. Your physician will take a medical and mental history and conduct a physical examination. If you have a physical or mental disorder, he or she will treat that disorder.

2. If you don't have another physical or mental illness, your physician will use your PMS/PMDD symptom charts to confirm your symptoms are consecutive and assess their severity. If your symptoms are mild to moderate, your doctor will recommend lifestyle and diet changes and ask you to wait two to three months to see how those changes affect your symptoms.

3. If lifestyle changes don't improve your symptoms, then your physician is likely to recommend that you try oral contraceptives or an SSRI.

4. If your symptoms are severe, the first course of action is usually an intermittent dose of an SSRI, such as Sarafem, along with recommended lifestyle changes, such as increasing exercise and reducing stress.

5. If you don't respond to the first drug, your doctor will likely recommend another SSRI, along with continued lifestyle changes.

6. At this point, after you have tried two different SSRIs, most physicians will recommend you consider cognitive-behavioral therapy to recognize negative thoughts and behaviors and replace them with positive ones or they will recommend low-dose anxiolytics, such as alprazolam (which can be addictive) during the luteal phase.

7. If anxiolytics and therapy fail to provide adequate relief, your doctor may suggest that you suppress your menstrual cycle using GnRH analogues or danazol for two or three menstrual cycles.

8. Surgical options are usually considered only if other treatment options have failed.

Chapter 13

Managing PMS

WOMEN TEND TO DREAD PMS not only because it affects them physically and emotionally, but because it makes them feel powerless. They feel they're at the mercy of a biological process. But PMS is manageable. How you feel before your period has a lot to do with the choices you make. There are good PMS-coping strategies, proven to help relieve your symptoms, and there are bad ones. Learn the strategies that can help ease your PMS experience and stop dreading the time before your period.

How to Live with PMS

You will have some 450 to 480 periods in your lifetime. Even if you don't experience PMS until your twenties or thirties, that still means you'll have between 200 and 300 periods preceded by days of pain, discomfort, and moodiness. That's too much time spent feeling bad—and since there's no miracle cure for PMS, the best you can do is to learn to live with it.

But living with PMS doesn't mean that you shouldn't seek treatment, far from it. Instead, think of it as a process in which you try different approaches to help relieve your discomfort. When something works, stick with it. When it doesn't, try something else. This can mean you adjust your diet, seek medical help, or try alternative treatments, like herbal supplements or acupuncture. But consult your doctor.

PMS is a collection of nearly 200 different symptoms. It's counterproductive to think there should be one solution for all of your symptoms, since there are multiple issues you need to address. Some symptoms will respond better to medication and others to lifestyle changes. Cutting back on salt in your diet may reduce your bloating, but it won't necessarily help your headaches or your nausea, and it's unlikely to reduce the number of arguments you have with your spouse, unless you're arguing about table salt or French fries! Similarly, choosing to go on antidepressants may dramatically relieve your mood symptoms, but it won't eliminate the sources of stress in your life that make you irritated or angry.

The Importance of Coping Strategies

Because PMS is an ongoing problem, most women develop a range of strategies to handle their symptoms. Over time, they've figured out that doing certain things and avoiding others makes the premenstrual phase more bearable: they may avoid their friends or seek their support, eat certain kinds of foods, take over-the-counter pain relievers, or call in sick to work.

Coping strategies, which are simply skills that we develop to respond to life situations, are varied and highly personal. What works for one woman may not work for another. But some strategies are better than others.

The Wrong Coping Strategies

How many times have you tried something that you knew didn't work particularly well just because you felt as though you had to do something? Or because you were more comfortable trying something familiar? Or because you'd run out of other things to try? These are just some of the reasons women turn time and again to things that only help deal with PMS in the short term, if they help at all. Some choices are more about ignoring PMS rather than dealing with it.

Essential

> If PMS is overwhelming you, consider therapy, which can teach you better coping strategies to deal with your symptoms, as well as with the sources of stress in your life.

Overeating

You feel lousy; you're bloated, depressed and discouraged. All you want to do is eat some ice cream, a big bowl of spaghetti, or some cheese pizza. PMS-induced food cravings for sweets, salt, and carbohydrates may be caused by low levels of serotonin. Some experts believe that women eat these foods as a way to regulate their moods. In other words, eating is self-medication. Whether the theory about food cravings and serotonin is accurate, giving in to cravings by stuffing yourself with these foods ultimately will make you feel worse. American culture is obsessed by appearance, often at the expense of health. Overeating is unhealthy, and it makes you feel bad about your supposed lack of control. It also has the potential to make your PMS much worse, since being overweight is a risk factor for getting PMS.

Focusing on Your Symptoms

Thinking about how bad your symptoms are is a surefire way to feel worse. A number of studies have shown that the more women know about PMS, the worse they feel. This may be because the knowledge legitimizes their experience; they always felt pain or discomfort but never attributed it to PMS. Or it may be because the women now pay attention to symptoms they had previously ignored. Constant negative thinking about PMS is a self-fulfilling prophecy: the more you think about how bad you feel, the worse you actually will feel. There's something to be said for looking on the bright side of things.

Taking It Out on Others or Yourself

Yes, you feel terrible, and yes, you want to lash out, but that strategy backfires as well. The people in your life—your spouse, siblings, children, friends—feel attacked and may become angry or fearful. They learn to avoid you. Meanwhile, even when you're in the grips of your worst PMS anger, there's usually a small part of you that realizes you're being unreasonable or acting out of proportion to the situation. So while yelling at your husband feels good or justified in the moment, it ultimately alienates him and makes you feel remorseful.

Yes, you have PMS and are sometimes mean to others. Stop beating yourself up about it! PMS is driven by biology. You're not a bad person because you yell at your spouse or your kids. If you feel as though you need to be perfect, PMS is sure to undermine your self-esteem when you inevitably fail at behaving as you think you should.

Avoiding Treatment

Telling yourself that you'll just have to live with your symptoms is one of the worst things you can do to yourself and your family. The symptoms you attribute to PMS may actually be caused by another disease. If you don't get it treated, you could be jeopardizing your health. Also, PMS symptoms take a toll on your body and over time can lead to serious health issues. For example, some women have PMS symptoms that begin at ovulation and persist through the end of their period, resulting in a three-week ordeal with only a one-week break between symptoms. Over time, they become so emotionally and physically exhausted from the PMS that the one-week break is not sufficient to rejuvenate and their symptoms begin to look like a chronic mood disorder. Getting treated in a case like this may provide some long-term relief.

Escaping

Some women are so bothered by their PMS symptoms they turn to alcohol, drugs, shopping, or overeating as a way of escaping. Don't let PMS drive you into habits that are self-destructive, unhealthy, and expensive. Other women have such significant emotional symptoms that they withdraw socially during their premenstrual phase. This too is potentially harmful because this kind of escapism cuts you off from the very people who can provide you with a support system that will help you better manage your PMS.

Pushing Yourself

Pushing yourself to achieve more in a given day or a week is a common way we deal with our stressful lives. You figure if you can just get this one errand, this one project, this one chore completed, then you could catch up on all the things you've let slip. But you never seem to catch up. It's similar with PMS. Many women try to live their normal lives even when they are physically or emotionally incapacitated. They think that they have to do everything they'd normally do, but this habit of pushing themselves beyond their abilities only leaves them feeling more stressed. Cut yourself a break and pamper yourself when you're feeling below par because of PMS.

Making Medications Your Lifeline

Medications, whether anti-inflammatories, diuretics, or antidepressants, can truly be helpful, but ultimately, they treat the symptoms, not the causes. Medical experts haven't figured out a way to treat the cause of PMS, short of menopause. Since medications are often so effective, however, you may be tempted to medicate your symptoms instead of adjusting your lifestyle to include exercise, changing your diet, or getting therapy, all of which can help you live a healthier, less stressful life.

The Right Coping Strategies

Although the right coping strategies are unlikely to make your PMS disappear, they can make the experience more bearable. They work, in part, because they make you feel more in control and introduce habits that enhance other aspects of your life.

Become Informed about Your Health

Knowing what causes PMS, learning what to expect each month, and finding ways to treat your symptoms is the best way to cope with PMS. It puts you in the driver's seat, it lets you prepare both physically and mentally for the experience, and it gives you options on how to treat PMS.

Take responsibility for your health, your habits, and your behaviors. It's one thing to acknowledge you have PMS; it's another thing entirely to blame your negative behaviors on your condition. If you take responsibility, you will be more motivated to learn new habits, introduce or increase exercise, and make better food choices.

Enlist the Support of Your Family and Friends

Teach them about PMS and how they can help you. For example, your family needs to be aware of your cycle, so they can prepare to make themselves scarce if they know you want to be left alone, and also so they know when to step in and give you a much-needed objective perspective if necessary. Research has shown that strong social support systems, including family closeness and connectedness, direct communication, and problem-focused family skills, are interconnected with overall health and wellness.

 Fact

A 2001 study in the *Journal of Applied Psychology* found that optimism and social support have a great effect on how much distress a person feels after a traumatic incident. Researchers studied rescue workers who responded at the crash of USAir 427, which crashed in Pennsylvania killing everyone aboard. The researchers found that those workers who were optimistic reported less distress, were more likely to use problem-focused coping strategies, and sought social support.

Friendships are an important part of a strong social support system, but if you have friends with PMS, they can provide you with an insider's perspective on PMS, and commiserate with you like no one else can. Finally, these friends can also share tips on coping and treatment that you might not be aware of since they are also dealing with similar symptoms.

Take It Easy

If you know your days are going to be stress-filled and challenging, don't overschedule or plan too much. Taking it easy will reduce stress and ease your symptoms.

You may have to work, or care for a child, or fulfill any one of a number of responsibilities, but taking a break of a few minutes during the days when your PMS is bad will give you both a physical and emotional respite.

Simple relaxation and breathing techniques can help introduce some calmness and sanity into your routine and into days when you are especially moody and irritable. Relaxation therapy can range from visualization techniques and deep-breathing exercises to home-grown versions, such as taking a warm bath surrounded by scented candles to hot stone massages (or warm gel packs for the less indulgent). You can also try practices like yoga, meditation, or prayer.

Recognize Negative Thought Patterns

During PMS, you may feel as though you're at the mercy of your symptoms, that there's nothing you can do, and that you might as well give up trying. Or maybe your bloating has caused your weight to soar and your self-esteem to plummet. Negative thought patterns in which you believe the worst possible scenario is the likeliest or generalize that everything is wrong simply because one thing did not go as planned are common in PMS. These patterns fuel your depression and anxiety and ultimately make you feel worse. You need to recognize the negative thoughts and replace them with positive ones. For women with severe PMS symptoms, cognitive and behavioral therapy can be very helpful, but for milder PMS symptoms, a family member or friend can often help give you some perspective on what's really going on.

Learn to Communicate

A lot of the anger and irritation women unleash during PMS is caused by poor communication skills. If you haven't learned to communicate well and tend to keep things bottled up, the two-week period when your hormones fluctuate and your mood is unstable provide a prime opportunity to lash out. Learning to be an effective communicator will help you confront your problems and teach you how to discuss them before they become so overwhelming that you burst out in an angry tirade.

Problem-Solve

Problem solving is a great tool in your arsenal to beat PMS. If you look at PMS as a great, inescapable problem, it leaves you helpless, but approaching it as a condition that you can treat gives you the ability to improve it.

Essential

Problem-focused coping strategies including changing your behavior, becoming informed about a stressful situation, and creating or joining support networks such as self-help groups. Emotion-focused coping strategies include avoiding thinking about a stressful situation, putting a positive spin on the situation, or wishing it were different.

Psychologists identify two general types of coping strategies: problem-focused and emotion-focused. People who use problem-focused strategies take action to minimize their stress, while those who use emotion-focused strategies try to minimize or eliminate the unpleasant emotions associated with the stressful situation. Take a problem-focused approach, but problem-solve in bits and pieces. Trying to get rid of all your symptoms simultaneously may be impossible. Start with what's bothering you the most and go from there.

Exercise

Exercise has tremendous health and emotional benefits: it can reduce your risk of heart disease, lower blood pressure, improve posture and back problems, and improve depression. Aerobic exercise increases levels of the neurotransmitters serotonin, dopamine, and norepinephrine and improves cognitive function, and even creativity! Any activity that elevates your heart rate—walking, jogging, swimming, tennis, or dancing—is beneficial. In addition, some exercises that focus on flexibility, such as yoga and Pilates, can also provide an aerobic workout if you do them with enough intensity. You'll know you're working out hard enough to get an aerobic benefit if it's difficult to carry on a conversation while you're exercising but not working so hard that you can't catch your breath.

 Alert

Increased levels of the hormone progesterone cause elevated breathing, which means your demand for oxygen rises during PMS. Also, before your period, your core body temperature usually rises, so your body has a more difficult time cooling off. Therefore during your period, exercise, but lessen the intensity and make sure you work out in a well-ventilated area, wear clothes that wick sweat away from your skin, and drink plenty of fluids.

Sleep

Many women have sleep problems during PMS, but inadequate or poor sleep can impair your short-term memory, judgment, your ability to process information, and your reaction times. You can improve sleep by eliminating distractions in your bedroom (i.e., no paperwork, computer, or television), keeping the temperature cool, and avoiding caffeine and alcohol in the evening and before bedtime. If you still can't get a good night's rest during PMS, consider taking quick power naps that last only twenty minutes or so; they have been proven to be restorative.

Eat Right

You can improve your PMS symptoms by choosing to eat healthful foods—fruits, vegetables, lean meats—and avoiding foods that are high in sugar, salt, or caffeine. In addition, choose foods that have beneficial effects on PMS, such as leafy green vegetables (collard greens, kale, and spinach) and dairy products, which are high in calcium, and soy-based foods, which contain isoflavones, (substances that have estrogen-like properties). (Chapters 16 and 17 discuss the dietary culprits that worsen PMS and provide recipes for healthy, PMS-friendly foods.)

Know Your Body

How well do you know your body? Do you know the ins and outs of your menstrual cycle? Are your cycle days consistent, or do they vary from month to month? Do you ovulate every month? How many days are in your follicular phase? What about your luteal phase? If you know the answers to these questions, you are way ahead of the game.

However, it's much more likely that you don't know these details. People tend to take their bodies for granted, especially if they have no major health issues that force them to pay attention. Women who take oral contraceptives have even less reason to chart the cycles because the packaging of their medications does that for them. They know exactly when to expect their period.

Yet knowing your body is an essential part of treating PMS. Medical diagnosis is an exercise in deduction: your doctor evaluates you, looks at your medical history, asks questions, maybe runs some tests, and, you hope, tells you what's wrong. But accurate diagnosis depends on good information. Not being able to provide that information will considerably extend the diagnostic process.

Let's say you go to your doctor because you get splitting headaches, bloating, indigestion, and mood swings during PMS. You want your doctor to suggest or maybe prescribe something at that visit. But when he or she asks you about your symptoms and when they occur in your cycle, you can only give general answers. Your doctors will probably ask you to chart your symptoms for a couple of months before going any further. Now the health problem you wanted to treat today has just been pushed back two months.

Keep a Menstrual Diary

Menstrual diaries are primarily used to track periods, fertility, or PMS symptoms. A basic menstrual diary notes when your period starts and ends, and when your next period begins, but you can make it as complex and detailed as you want.

To start, you need only a monthly wall or desk calendar. Simply mark the days of your period and note any days when you have discharge or pain.

If you want more detail about your cycle, such as when you ovulate, add it to your PMS diary. For example, if your cycle is very erratic, veering from sixteen days to forty days down to twenty-five, you might not be ovulating during every cycle. You can track ovulation using your menstrual diary. All you have to do is take your basal body temperature every morning and write it down on your calendar. After three or four months, a pattern will emerge that can help you figure out if and when you ovulate.

Your menstrual diary should include the following information:

- What day did your period start?
- What day did it end?
- Did you feel any pain associated with your period?
- How many tampons did you use each day?
- Did you notice any discharge? When?

- Did you miss work or social activities? On which days?
- Did you take any medications for cramping or other symptoms?
- Did you have any side effects or reactions to the medication?
- Any other information that is relevant.

Keep a PMS Diary

A PMS diary is a more detailed version of a menstrual diary, primarily focused on your symptoms and their effects. In addition to noting the days you have your period, write down your physical and emotional symptoms, their severity, and indicate whether you took any medications to relieve them, as well as any side effects you experienced.

 Fact

A group in the United Kingdom, the National Association for Pre-menstrual Syndrome, developed an interactive menstrual chart that allows users to record their symptoms and their severity and to track them over time. In addition, perimenopausal women can identify and monitor the change in their symptoms and track their frequency or severity. It is available at *www.pms.org.uk*.

Your PMS diary should record:

Physical symptoms
- Bloating
- Breast swelling/tenderness
- Muscle or joint pain
- Headaches
- Sleep problems
- Increase or decrease in sexual interest

- Acne
- Indigestion, constipation, or diarrhea
- Fatigue
- Cramping

Cognitive symptoms

- Trouble concentrating
- Trouble remembering
- Clumsiness

Emotional symptoms

- Depression
- Anxiety
- Anger
- Mood swings
- Aggression
- Social withdrawal

Medications (whether or not used to treat PMS)

- NSAIDs, such as ibuprofen
- Diuretics
- Herbal supplements
- Prescription drugs
- Vitamins, dietary supplements
- Medication side effects/reactions
- How the medications make you feel

You can create a homemade version of a menstrual diary or choose a preprinted one. There are multiple versions of premenstrual calendars available online or through your doctor. Some Web sites have blank calendars that you can print out or download, or even let you track your symptoms online.

CHAPTER 14

The Mind-Body Connection

EMOTIONAL AND PHYSICAL WELL-BEING are inextricably linked: poor emotional health weakens your immune system and can cause physical pain, while physical pain often has emotional consequences, such as depression. So when you're suffering from PMS, do you address the physical symptoms and hope that improves your emotional health? Or do you see a counselor and hope it improves your physical symptoms? Do you see a therapist? An obstetrician-gynecologist? Both?

A Complicated Relationship

Your body responds to how you think and feel; in effect, there's a connection between your mind and your body. If you're depressed and anxious, your body aches too.

PMS illustrates this dynamic perfectly. Not only does premenstrual syndrome include both physical and mood symptoms, its cyclical pattern means that even as you start to feel better with the onset of your period, the knowledge that you'll experience your symptoms again in a few weeks can make you stressed, depressed, and anxious. This sets the stage for an exhausting pattern: The more you dread PMS, the worse you actually feel.

Understanding the mind-body connection in PMS is important because it will help you understand if there is something besides PMS at work. It will also help target the type of treatment. For example, if your lifestyle or personal situation is highly stressful—because of work, a life change like divorce, financial problems, or other problems—treating PMS with medications may help, but relieving the source of the stress will help more.

⌴ Essential

Stressful events, as well as depression and anxiety, can cause a host of physical symptoms including appetite changes (either overeating or a loss of appetite), chest pains, constipation, diarrhea, headaches, fatigue, back pain, high blood pressure, shortness of breath, palpitations, and sexual problems.

Yet this is where it gets tricky. Doctors, often the first health-care professionals women with PMS turn to, are great at diagnosing and treating medical problems. Unfortunately, they're not necessarily the best authorities on the psychological and social aspects, and PMS is more than a medical problem. It has a full complement of mood symptoms, some of which are better addressed by a psychologist or even a psychiatrist, and it is exacerbated by lifestyle issues such as poor diet and lack of exercise. Even your OB-GYN may not ultimately be the best PMS expert for you, although he or she is probably your best first point of contact when seeking help. How do you know if you should see a doctor or a psychologist? Should you go into therapy? Or should you join a self-help group? Maybe you should see a nutritionist to improve your diet or get involved in an exercise program instead. As you navigate your treatment options, consider which symptoms are more bothersome or painful, and let that help guide your treatment.

Different Types of Treatment

On the Internet, you can find a PMS "expert" at the drop of a hat, but in real life, it is considerably harder. All sorts of medical and non-medical professionals treat premenstrual syndrome: primary care physicians, OB-GYNs, nurse practitioners, psychologists, counselors, psychiatrists, chiropractors, and nutritionists among them. Predictably, depending on their education and philosophy, each of these "experts" treats PMS differently.

There are some critical differences, however. Primary care physicians, gynecologists, and psychiatrists can prescribe drugs to treat your PMS symptoms, as can nurse practitioners. But psychologists cannot. Therapists and counselors both focus on therapy, but therapists don't all approach personal issues the same way, nor do they all have the same training. Finally, there are a number of treatments for PMS-related issues outside of medication and therapy, such as relieving stress and painful physical symptoms by adjusting the body's musculoskeletal systems through chiropractic care.

Therapy, Medicine, or Both?

If you suffer from severe emotional symptoms during PMS, psychotherapy may be the best treatment option. But therapy can also help you with the physical aspects of PMS by helping uncover the emotional issues at the root of your headaches, digestive problems, or backache. Professionals who practice psychotherapy include psychologists, psychiatrists, social workers, and counselors. Each of these professionals has different licensing requirements and different areas of expertise.

Question

What is psychotherapy?
Psychotherapy is a technique designed to improve a person's physical and mental health function. Therapy and psychotherapy are often used interchangeably to describe this process. Generally, psychotherapy consists of conversations between a therapist and a client/patient—this is the reason psychotherapy is sometimes referred to as "talk therapy"—but it can also include supportive dialogue, sensory stimulation, and cognitive-behavioral approaches.

The therapist's job is to help you recognize and cope with your negative mood symptoms, understand why they occurred, and help prevent them from reoccurring in the future. Patients are required to be honest and involved during their sessions. Therapy offers a lot of potential to recognize the root causes that worsen your symptoms, but it can take time to resolve core problems. In contrast, physicians may be able to find medical causes for your emotional symptoms and prescribe medications that provide immediate relief. Consider which approach has more long-term benefit for you.

Seeing a Psychologist

Psychologists are mental health specialists who help individuals resolve personal and emotional matters. Usually, psychologists earn a doctoral degree (Ph.D. or Psy.D.) in psychology and have undergone clinical training. They offer counseling focused on normal developmental issues, everyday stress, phobias, depression, and issues resulting from abuse.

Unlike psychiatrists, most psychologists are not medical doctors and are unable to prescribe drugs. However, they have years of training and experience in understanding human behavior, emotions, and mental processes. Psychologists can work for a university, a clinic, or a business, or they can be in individual practice.

All Psychologists Are Not Alike

There are three main branches in psychology: cognitive, behavioral, and dynamic. The right one for you depends on your symptoms, as well as on your comfort level with treatment techniques.

Cognitive psychology studies the mental processes underlying behavior and examines areas such as perception, learning, problem solving, memory, attention, language, and emotions. In other words, cognitive therapists are interested in how people understand, diagnose, and solve problems; in treatment, they tend to look at dysfunction and difficulties arising from irrational or faulty thinking.

Behavioral psychology, or behaviorism, looks at how behavior results from interactions with the environment and from internal stimuli. Behavioral therapists look at problems as the result of how their clients have been conditioned over the years, rather than as the result of an internal mental state.

Dynamic psychology looks at issues that begin in early childhood but continue to motivate the person in adulthood on an unconscious level. Sigmund Freud's work on dream interpretation, in which dreams are manifestations of unconscious thoughts, is a classic example of this branch of psychology.

Research has shown that cognitive therapy seems to work better with depression, while behavioral therapy is useful for breaking unwanted habits, such as smoking, overcoming phobias (through desensitization), and stopping negative thought patterns. Beyond that, however, no other differences regarding effectiveness have been found among the different therapeutic approaches. In fact, many psychologists now combine therapeutic approaches to treat their patients. Ultimately, if you want to try therapy to work on problems that appear or appear worse during PMS, the choice of psychologist is up to you.

Psychology is a very broad field, and it includes different approaches to the study of mental processes and behavior. Here are some specializations:

- **Clinical psychology** is used to treat mental distress; clinical psychologists assess mental health problems, and conduct and use scientific research to understand mental health.
- **Development psychology** is the scientific study of progressive psychological changes that occur in people as they change.
- **Health psychology** uses psychological principles to promote health and prevent illness.
- **Medical psychology** treats the body and the mind as interconnected. Medical psychologists are trained in the biological aspects of mental illness as it relates to physical illness.

- **Popular psychology** includes concepts and theories that explain human behavior and mental processes that are not drawn from the technical field of psychology. Popular psychology offers insights into human behavior, but its findings are not supported by systematic analysis.

Finding a Psychologist

There are several resources to help you find a psychologist. The American Psychological Association has an online referral service (*www.apa.org*), as does the National Register of Health Service Providers in Psychology, a nonprofit organization that credentials psychologists (*www.findapsychologist.org*). In addition, your health plan may provide a list of mental care providers, and hospitals in your community can provide referrals or may even have premenstrual clinics with therapists on staff.

Other Mental Health Professionals

Psychiatrists, counselors, and social workers also provide therapy. But their training and the types of patients or clients they work with vary.

Psychiatrists are licensed medical doctors who specialize in diagnosing, treating, and preventing mental and emotional disorders such as clinical depression, bipolar disorder, schizophrenia, and anxiety disorders. They can provide both psychotherapy and drug therapy. Psychiatric treatment is most appropriate for women with PMDD and individuals with other mental or mood disorders.

Not every clinician who practices psychiatry is necessarily a licensed medical doctor. Some others are nurse practitioners, medical psychologists, and physician assistants. Psychiatric physicians (psychiatrists), nurse practitioners, and medical psychologists are all trained in the biology of mental illness and can provide the same treatment.

What does a mental health professional look at when working with women with PMS or PMDD symptoms? Typically, he or she will conduct a psychiatric evaluation that focuses on the symptoms of depression, seasonal affective disorder, alcohol and drug use, early victimization and trauma, family history of affective disorder, alcoholism, and current stressors. In this way, the therapist can distinguish what other issues are potentially affecting the client's mood.

 Alert

Not every medical professional who practices psychiatry can prescribe drugs. Medical psychologists, who have specialized training in clinical psychopharmacology (the use of psychiatric drugs), are not usually allowed to prescribe medications. Only two states, Louisiana and New Mexico, allow medical psychologists to prescribe drugs. Nurse practitioners generally provide short-term psychotherapy, conduct physical assessments, and can prescribe drugs.

Seeing a Counselor

Mental health counselors diagnose and treat mental health problems, as well as offer psychotherapy, crisis management, and alcohol or substance abuse treatment. Licensed counselors usually have a master's degree in counseling, at least two years' clinical work supervised by a certified mental health profession after their master's degree, and have passed a state or national licensure exam. Their training is comparable to clinical social workers and marriage and family therapists.

Counselors may work with individuals, couples, families, and children. They offer a collaborative, supporting, engaged, and non-judgmental relationship to their client. Their job is to listen and reflect (but they will become more involved in cases of serious and imminent danger).

Counselors offer brief and solution-focused therapy, rather than intense psychotherapy.

Although they don't have as much formal training as psychologists or psychiatrists, counselors may be the perfect choice for women whose emotional and mood-related PMS symptoms stem from problems communicating, family or personal issues, substance-abuse problems, marital problems, or stressful work situations—issues that can be more quickly resolved than serious emotional or mental disorders.

Counselors lead group counseling sessions and offer stress management groups (e.g., biofeedback, relaxation training) and individual counseling. Many PMS support groups offered by community health organizations or hospitals are run by counselors. For these reasons, counselors tend to be more accessible and affordable than psychologists or psychiatrists.

 Fact

According to the October 2000 issue of *Psychotherapy Finances*, a newsletter for behavioral health practitioners, the median cost per session for mental health counselors is $85. In comparison, the median cost per session for psychologists is $100; for psychiatrists, it is $145.

The cost of therapy doesn't have to be a deterrent if you want to explore treatments for PMS. Many psychologists, therapists, and psychiatrists offer a sliding scale to patients who can't afford to pay the full fees for therapy. The reduced fees are usually based on family income. In addition, many companies offer employee assistance programs that provide counseling for personal problems. Finally, if your employer offers health insurance, the insurance may cover some mental health treatment.

Seeing a Doctor

While the majority of women don't seek help for their PMS, those who do usually see their doctor—either a primary care provider or obstetrician-gynecologist—first. Unfortunately, this is often the beginning of a long road. Medical treatment is not the quick solution many people assume. One study showed that it took more than five years on average for women to get their symptoms diagnosed as PMS! When your doctor treats your PMS, he or she first eliminates other possible physical causes of the symptoms and then suggests lifestyle changes before finally prescribing medications.

The upside to seeing your doctor is that you already have an established relationship with each other, and he or she probably has a pretty good version of your medical history (possibly even a complete medical history), which can help narrow the medical possibilities for your symptoms in the initial stages of diagnosis. Your doctor can diagnose you with PMS or PMDD and can prescribe medications and discuss diet and lifestyle changes.

The downside is that he or she may not be trained to address emotional issues or to counsel patients. If this is the case, your doctor will look at you from a medical perspective not from the perspective of a counselor, so in effect, you may be only getting half the treatment you require. So while these primary care physicians and ob-gyns have a great deal of medical expertise, unless they have a special interest in PMS, they aren't necessarily experts in the field of PMS treatment, since the symptoms are so broad and still so little understood. Such OB-GYNs, whose patients are exclusively women, aren't necessarily PMS experts, especially in regard to the emotional or mood symptoms. So it is important that you talk to your doctor about his or her areas of expertise and experience dealing with PMS to determine if you need additional consultation.

Prescribing for PMS

What do doctors prescribe for PMS? A few years ago, it may have been progesterone; today it may also be an SSRI. One retrospective survey published in the journal *BMC Women's Health* found that

that, at least in the United Kingdom, PMS remedies have changed over the years.

In 2002, several U.K. researchers reviewed physician prescribing patterns between 1993 and 1998 using a database that contained the medical records of more than 282,000 women, 5,891 of whom were diagnosed with PMS. They found that despite little evidence that supports their effectiveness, progestins were the most widely prescribed treatment for PMS, accounting for 40 percent of all prescriptions. Vitamin B6 accounted for 22 percent of prescriptions in 1993 but dropped to 11 percent between 1997 and 1998. Selective serotonin reuptake inhibitors only accounted for 2 percent of prescriptions in 1993 but rose to 16 percent by 1998, the second most-common treatment. Overall, the study showed a yearly decrease in the number of prescriptions linked to diagnoses for PMS.

It appears that despite its lack of evidence, progesterone enjoys a halo effect as a PMS treatment. The study researchers note that Katharina Dalton, a pioneering British gynecologist and endocrinologist who coined the term *premenstrual syndrome* and was instrumental in PMS becoming a recognized disorder, was a vocal proponent of progesterone for many years.

The study also found that prescription-linked diagnoses of PMS fell fourfold between 1993 and 1998. In other words, fewer women either were being diagnosed with PMS or did not receive prescriptions for their PMS.

Sifting Through Your Choices

Now that you know a bit about the different approaches OB-GYNs, primary care physicians, psychologists, psychiatrists, and counselors bring to PMS treatment, here are some factors to help you decide which type of health-care provider may be best for you.

See a primary care provider
- If you go to your PCP for gynecological exams
- If you have other health issues besides PMS, such as diabetes or irritable bowel syndrome

- If you are interested in trying prescription medications

See an OB-GYN
- If you use your OB-GYN as your primary doctor
- If you are more comfortable talking with someone who works exclusively with women
- If you are interested in trying prescription medications

See a counselor
- If you want to improve family relationships or communication skills
- If you want to resolve a particular troubling situation
- If you want to learn how to reduce stress
- If you are interested in participating in a group environment

See a psychologist
- If you have disabling emotional or mood symptoms
- If you are interested in talk therapy
- If you want to establish a long-term relationship with a therapist

See a psychiatrist
- If you have disabling emotional or mood symptoms
- If you suspect you may have another mental health disorder
- If you are interested in drug therapy

Treating Yourself

The majority of women don't go to doctors, psychologists, or even counselors. They self-treat their PMS. This can mean anything from adopting a "suck it up" attitude, in which you steadfastly ignore your symptoms until you get your period, to taking some Motrin, grabbing a hot water bottle, and spending a night watching sappy movies, to overhauling your diet and trying herbal supplements. Although these strategies may do the trick for PMS-related physical symptoms, they're not likely to reduce PMS-related mood symptoms.

In the first place, it's difficult to recognize the signs that you're overreacting or responding inappropriately to a given situation. Any woman in the midst of an angry tirade because her husband or boyfriend expects her to pick up the dry cleaning, cook dinner, and clean up afterward is not going to stop in the middle to think, "I have PMS." It's more likely she'll yell and rage and feel justified in doing so, until, at some point after the argument, it may dawn on her that she's overreacted.

Second, it's tough to self-treat mood symptoms, especially if you don't recognize them. There aren't any pills that you can take to reduce stress, improve your coping skills, or learn to be a better communicator.

However, there are several stress-reduction strategies you might try. Stress-reduction techniques—such as learning to control your breathing, using imagery to relax yourself, and positive thinking—can be very helpful. So can massage, listening to music, exercise, or reducing or eliminating the factors that cause your stress.

You can try environmental, physical, and mental techniques to reduce stress. Environmental techniques include listening to music or relaxation tapes, adjusting lighting and temperature, and removing sources of distraction, such as computers or television, to create a calming environment. Another environmental technique is to prepare for a potentially stressful event or interaction by asking for instructions, direction, or feedback or rehearsing a dialogue or conversation.

Physical techniques include breathing control (such as the deep-breathing methods practiced in yoga), biofeedback (a technique in which you learn to control stress by using electronic sensors that are attached to your body), and physical exercise.

Mental stress-reduction techniques include practicing positive thinking, using imagery to relax yourself, and even self-hypnosis.

Chapter 15

Self-Care for PMS

SELF-CARE, ESPECIALLY NUTRITION AND EXERCISE, can signifi-cantly reduce and temporarily ease the pain of PMS symptoms. Self-care strategies include taking magnesium and calcium, changing your diet, exercising regularly, enlisting the support of others, using over-the-counter medication, and taking herbal supplements. Some self-care methods are simple daily adjustments and others require lifestyle changes. Difficult or not, however, making the necessary changes is worth it.

Exercise

Yes, you should exercise, but then you've always heard that, right? It still doesn't make it easier to do. If you're usually sedentary, incorpo-rating exercise into your schedule can sound like an overwhelming life change. Even if you're reasonably active, stepping up your exer-cise program can be hard, often because of time constraints or other perceived barriers. But the myriad health benefits of exercise, as well as its potential to relieve PMS symptoms, are worth the investment.

Moderate exercise can have a dramatic effect on your overall well-being. Exercise helps lower blood pressure and cholesterol, reduces your risk of heart disease, helps prevent osteoporosis, helps protect you from certain cancers, improves your strength and mobil-ity, and helps you lose and maintain weight. Research shows that exercise can also reduce your PMS symptoms.

Exercise, especially aerobic exercise, increases the release of beta-endorphin, a neurotransmitter that boosts the immune system, kills cancer cells, and acts as an analgesic to numb or dull pain. One 1991 study showed that aerobic exercise caused beta-endorphin levels to rise fivefold over normal levels. This rise seems to be unrelated to the amount of athletic training a person has (although athletes seem to metabolize beta-endorphins more efficiently), while the duration and intensity of the exercise does have an effect on how much beta-endorphin levels rise.

Exercise also impacts hormone levels. One study showed that forty-minute sessions of resistance or endurance exercise significantly increased blood levels of estrogen, testosterone, and growth hormones in women who exercised compared with women who did not. Exercise counteracts the estrogen and endorphin withdrawal that happens in the luteal phase of your menstrual cycle and depresses progesterone levels. In other words, it appears to control the hormonal imbalance associated with PMS.

The link between exercise and PMS has not been effectively studied, but despite this, experts commonly recommend exercise as a treatment for women with PMS and PMDD. Researchers do know that women who are active seem to have fewer PMS symptoms. For example, female athletes are less likely to have PMS. Research has also shown that exercise has a beneficial effect on a number of specific PMS symptoms such as migraine and depression. Yet even with all its health benefits, many people resist exercise or have trouble sustaining an exercise program. If you suffer from PMS, it's important to try to counter these obstacles. Since exercise can ease depression, anxiety, and stress, and make you more physically fit, isn't it worth trying?

Exercise and Stress

Exercise is known to reduce stress, a major risk factor for PMS. Women who are stressed and also have strong PMS appear to use exercise as a coping mechanism for their symptoms. A 2004 study published in the *Journal of Women's Health* assessed 114 women between the ages of eighteen and thirty-three according to their PMS symptoms, quality of life, and exercise. Results showed that women with high PMS had significantly more stress and a poorer quality of life than women with low PMS. The relationship with exercise was more complicated. Women who said they exercised sometimes had more stress than women who exercised often or never. The researchers speculated that women with the worst PMS symptoms respond by exercising, while women who exercise often or never exercise don't associate exercise with their symptoms.

A 1999 telephone survey of 874 women in Virginia, published in the *Archives of Family Medicine*, also showed that women with PMS turn to exercise. The study showed that women with PMS were 2.9 times more likely to be physically active than women without PMS. Researchers recommended more study to determine if women with PMS exercise more regularly than women without PMS because they believe exercise is effective in managing their symptoms.

 ## Fact

PMS affects more than your body. It hurts your quality of life and your ability to work. Researchers at UCLA's Cedars-Sinai Health System found that women with PMS had reduced work productivity, experienced interference with hobbies, and missed a greater number of days of work for health reasons.

Exercise and Migraines

Since it increases endorphin levels, which have an analgesic effect, aerobic exercise reduces migraines. People with a history of migraines who participated in an aerobic exercise program experienced fewer migraines. Their migraines were also shorter and less intense, according to one study. Another study in which participants exercised three times a week for six weeks for forty minutes (a ten-minute warm-up, twenty minutes of exercise, followed by a ten-minute cooldown) showed that after four weeks, the participants' endorphin levels increased and their migraines were significantly reduced.

Exercise and Depression

More than one hundred studies have been conducted on exercise and depression, and the results consistently show that exercise boosts mood, increases energy level, and has a calming effect.

Exercise appears to be at least as effective as more traditional therapies for depression. A 1990 study by T. C. North and colleagues, published in *Exercise and Sports Medicine Reviews*, found that exercise produced effects comparable to psychotherapy and relieved depression more than either relaxation therapy or enjoyable activities. A 1997 study of clinically depressed individuals found that exercise produced the same effects as psychotherapy, behavioral interventions, and social contact.

Exercise and Anxiety

There is very strong evidence that exercise also reduces anxiety, another common PMS symptom. A 1991 study published in the journal *Sports Medicine* showed that people feel less anxious immediately after exercise, and this effect continues for the next several hours.

Several reviews of studies conducted between 1960 and 1995 on anxiety and exercise showed that both ongoing exercise programs and exercise performed for relatively short periods have an antianxiety effect. It didn't matter if the study subjects were anxious types, prone to anxiety on a regular basis, or if they were only anxious in very specific situations—they all benefited.

You'll achieve greater benefits depending on the type of exercise you do, how long you do it, and how anxious or fit you are. Aerobic exercise such as running, swimming, or cycling is better at reducing anxiety than non-aerobic exercise (e.g., strength-flexibility training). In addition, if your exercise training program is at least ten weeks long (and preferably longer than fifteen weeks), and if you are either highly anxious (such as panic disorder patients) or have a lower level of fitness, you'll see a greater anti-anxiety effect from exercise.

Other Benefits of Exercise

Exercise helps you live longer. One study conducted by the Cooper Institute for Aerobic Research in Dallas and published in the *Journal of the American Medical Association* found that a relatively modest amount of exercise affects mortality rates. Data from an eight-year study of 13,344 people showed that the higher the fitness level, the lower the death rate. The study subjects were grouped by gender into five groups, ranging from least to most fit. Women in the least-fit category had death rates 4.6 times higher than women in the most-fit category. The least-fit men had death rates 3.4 times higher than the most-fit men. The study showed that as little as thirty minutes of brisk walking was enough to drop the death rate by 60 percent for men and 48 percent for women.

Exercise also helps cut your risk for dementia. A 2006 study in the *Annals of Internal Medicine* showed that people who exercise three times a week or more are 30 percent to 40 percent less likely to develop Alzheimer's disease and other types of dementia.

 Fact

PMS costs! Researchers at UCLA's Cedars-Sinai Medical Center calculate that PMS costs $4,392 per year in direct medical costs, missed workdays, and lost productivity. In the 2005 study, researchers collected data on 374 women aged eighteen to forty-five. Administrative health claims data showed that PMS cost $59 in direct costs each year and $4,333 in indirect costs, such as missed workdays and lost productivity.

Social Support

A number of studies have found that women who have supportive spouses, friends, or family are better able to cope with the stress that causes many PMS symptoms. They also have a better perception of PMS.

For example, a small study of twenty-eight women in 1999 found participation in a peer support group that positively reframed the PMS experience reduced negative symptoms and also increased the women's personal resources. In other words, women who had peer support were able to see the bright side of PMS and, as a result, felt better and more in control.

In 1994, roughly at the time that PMDD was being added to the *DSM-IV*, Australian psychologist Elizabeth Harding argued that a lot of the emotional mood swings and poor job performance attributed to PMS were really caused by poor social interactions. Harding had 101 women fill out daily health and stress diaries for ten weeks and found that 18 percent occasionally showed marked premenstrual mood changes. But their mood changes were not all that different from those felt by non-menstruating women. Harding concluded that many women—one-quarter of those she studied—were chronically unhappy, felt they had little social support, had few coping skills, and felt their life was controlled by chance. Harding argued that rather than blaming PMS, the women needed to learn coping skills, relaxation strategies, stress management, and assertiveness training in order to feel better.

Boost Your Diet

Besides exercise, diet is the other big element in your life that is both controllable and has a major effect on how you feel during the premenstrual phase. It's no secret that in general, Americans eat very poorly with diets high in fat, carbohydrates, and calories. Americans depend heavily on processed foods rather than on fresh fruits and vegetables, fiber, and protein and often lack the essential vitamins and minerals that are found in unprocessed foods.

Is there a quick fix? Some people certainly think so. The dietary supplement industry is enormous, and so is the pharmaceutical industry. In the first case, "natural" herbs and supplements are touted to improve health and nutrition, and in the second, the symptoms of generally unhealthful lifestyles can be medicated.

Does this broad generalization apply to everyone? Of course not. There is a place for both supplements and pharmaceuticals, but a healthful and balanced diet is the crux of the matter.

For PMS, that means eating more fruits and vegetables, unprocessed cereals and grains, lean meat, fish, low-fat milk and dairy products, and margarine or oils rich in polyunsaturated fatty acids and vitamin E. It also means cutting back on caffeine, sodium, and alcohol, while boosting calcium, vitamin B6, and magnesium. Some women with PMS swear that replacing dairy with soy products and even taking evening primrose oil (to increase the intake of omega-6, a fatty acid essential to health) makes a huge difference in their symptoms. (Chapters 16 and 17 discuss PMS diet dos and don'ts in more detail and Chapter 17 has recipes for foods that are PMS-friendly.)

L. Essential

A 2001 study examined 144 overweight women who kept diet diaries over two menstrual cycles. When researchers analyzed the women's diaries, they found that women with PMS showed a significantly greater intake of carbohydrates and more "episodes of eating" during the premenstrual phase. Women without PMS did not show a difference in how much they ate premenstrually or postmenstrually.

Smoking

Smoking is bad for your health, but there also appears to be a connection between smoking and PMS. Studies suggest that cigarette smoking raises levels of prolactin, a hormone that can reduce progesterone levels. In this way, it can increase the severity of PMS symptoms. Smoking can also damage the reproductive system: the nicotine in cigarettes can damage ovaries, cause menstrual abnormalities, and decrease the production of estrogen. A 1999 study by researchers at the University of California, San Diego, found that cigarette smoking was associated with a host of menstrual irregularities:

an increased risk of bleeding between periods, excessively frequent periods, periods that lasted longer than one week, and irregular periods. In addition, women who smoke tend to go through menopause earlier.

Does PMS Make You Smoke More?

Smokers often use cigarettes to control anxiety, so women with strong PMS symptoms might smoke more during PMS. Researchers have looked at the connection between smoking and menstrual phase and the results are decidedly mixed.

For example, there's a strong association between smoking and a diagnosis of PMDD, but this is not necessarily because smoking causes PMDD, but because PMDD is a mood disorder similar to depression. Research has shown there's a strong correlation between smoking and a lifetime prevalence of depression. So in this case, it's the depressive disorder and not the menstrual aspect of PMDD that appears linked to smoking.

In another example, a 2000 study published in the journal *Addictive Behaviors* supported earlier findings that women with severe menstrual symptoms had more severe smoking abstinence effects, such as cravings and withdrawal symptoms, but menstrual phase did not appear to influence the desire for smoking.

Smoking is especially dangerous if you are taking oral contraceptives (whether to reduce PMS symptoms or to prevent pregnancy). Smoking increases your risk of developing cardiovascular problems such as blood clots; it also increases your risk of heart attacks and strokes. The risk increases as you age and with heavy smoking (fifteen or more cigarettes a day). The risks are significant in women over thirty-five. If you are a smoker over the age of thirty-five, you should not take oral contraceptives.

Vitamin B6

Vitamin B6 is commonly recommended as a PMS treatment, but there's only limited evidence to support that recommendation, at least as far as standardized medicine is concerned. In addition, too much vitamin B6 has some potentially serious side effects.

 Fact

Vitamin B is a complex of several vitamins that includes B1(thiamin), B2 (riboflavin), B6 (pyridoxine), B9 (folic acid), B12 (cyanocobalamin), pantothenic acid, and biotin. Although it was once thought to be a single vitamin, research showed that vitamin B was a complex of chemically distinct vitamins. As a result, the name shifted from vitamin B to the B vitamins or to B complex.

On the plus side, vitamin B6 may relieve breast pain and tenderness and PMS-related depression, while vitamin B6 and magnesium supplements may relieve PMS-related anxiety. On the minus side, high doses of the vitamin can lead to sensory neuropathy, a condition in which a person feels pain and numbness in the extremities and may even have difficulty walking. However, these effects only occur in doses that exceed 1,000 milligrams a day, and all evidence of negative effects are from vitamin B6 supplements not from food sources. Because of its potential toxic effects, the recommended maximum dose is 100 milligrams daily.

 Alert

Many natural supplement retailers sell vitamin B6 in high dosage packages. Some also recommend that women with PMS take between 100 and 200 milligrams in the two weeks before their periods. Women taking higher doses of vitamin B6 may experience side effects such as nausea, vomiting, and headache.

In 1990, researchers reviewed twelve studies in which vitamin B6 was compared to a placebo (neither study participants nor researchers knew who was taking the vitamin or the placebo) and concluded that evidence of a beneficial effect was weak.

A British review of twenty-five studies (sixteen of which were excluded because of poor or marginal quality) that together involved 940 women found that vitamin B6 was up to twice as effective as a placebo in relieving PMS. The study, published in the *British Medical Journal,* also found that very high doses, such as 600 milligrams, were no more beneficial than lower doses. The investigators recommend women start with a dose of 50 milligrams a day and take no more than 100 milligrams per day. However, they also stressed that because none of the studies they'd reviewed were randomized controlled trials (the gold standard of clinical testing), they could not definitively conclude the vitamin B6 was effective in treating PMS.

Food Sources of Vitamin B6

A balanced diet will provide you with enough vitamin B6. On average, women in the United States get 1.5 milligrams of vitamin B6 from the foods they consume. In contrast, the recommended dietary allowance is 1.3 milligrams for adult women aged nineteen to fifty. However, because some plant foods contain a type of vitamin B6 called pyridoxine glucoside, which is absorbed and used by the body only half as well as other forms of the vitamin, women may still need to boost their intake of foods rich in vitamin B6. The following foods are good sources: whole-grain cereals, bananas, potatoes, bell peppers, turnip greens, nuts, turkey, liver, avocados, green beans, chicken, spinach, and salmon. Strict vegetarians may need to eat foods fortified with vitamin B6 or take supplements to ensure they don't develop a nutritional deficiency.

Essential

Even though some foods contain more than the recommended dietary allowance of vitamin B6, only about 75 percent of it is "bio-available" or usable to the body.

Calcium

Calcium is good for more than your bones; it can also help to relieve PMS symptoms. A June 2005 study published in the *Archives of Internal Medicine* showed that a diet rich in calcium and vitamin D helps women reduce symptoms of PMS. It also suggests that calcium, combined with enough vitamin D, may help prevent PMS altogether.

Researchers looked at the dietary habits of more than 2,100 women, comparing the 1,057 who had PMS and the 1,068 who did not. They found that women who got the vitamin D equivalent of at least seven cups of milk—or 706 international units per day (or nearly twice the recommended daily allowance)—were 40 percent less likely to have PMS symptoms than women who got the equivalent of one cup or less of milk, 100 international units per day. Women who got the vitamin D equivalent of four and a half cups of milk, or about one and half times the recommended daily allowance, were 30 percent less likely to suffer from PMS. Experts recommend a daily dose of 400 international units of Vitamin D, however, the results of this study suggests women might benefit from twice that dose.

 Fact

Calcium supplements can be found either as separate, stand-alone supplements, or combined with magnesium. Vitamin D promotes calcium absorption, and both vitamin D and calcium are found in dairy products such as milk.

Magnesium

Magnesium is an essential nutrient that increases calcium absorption, which means it boosts the beneficial effects of calcium on PMS. Its other functions include regulating muscle contraction and relaxation, regulating blood sugar levels, promoting normal blood pressure, and playing a role in energy metabolism.

A 1999 study in the *Journal of Women's Health* found that 200 milligrams a day of magnesium reduced mild PMS-induced fluid retention, breast tenderness, and bloating by 40 percent. The researchers, who administered either a placebo or a magnesium supplement to study participants over two menstrual cycles, found there was no difference between the magnesium and the placebo in the first month. In the second month, however, women taking the magnesium had a greater reduction in symptoms.

Studies support magnesium's beneficial effect on PMS. For example, a 1998 study in the *American Journal of Obstetrics and Gynecology* found that 1,200 milligrams a day of chewable calcium carbonate reduced PMS symptoms such as water retention, food cravings, and pain by 48 percent, while placebo relieved symptoms by only 30 percent. The investigators concluded that "calcium supplementation is a simple and effective treatment in premenstrual syndrome, resulting in a major reduction in overall luteal phase symptoms."

There is also some evidence that magnesium supplementation may reduce the frequency and severity of migraine headaches. Two placebo-controlled studies demonstrated a beneficial effect on migraine, while another placebo-controlled study found no benefit compared to placebo.

Foods high in magnesium include buckwheat, nuts, and whole grains, as well as collard greens, dandelion greens, avocados, sweet corn, cheddar cheese, sunflower seeds, shrimp, dried fruit (figs, apricots, and prunes), and many other common fruits and vegetables.

CHAPTER 16

The PMS Diet

IF YOU GET BLOATED, irritable, and anxious, experience pounding headaches and indigestion, or suffer from sleep problems during PMS, your diet may be partly to blame. Target your symptoms by making some changes in how you eat. Feeling better doesn't necessarily require a diet overhaul—just some awareness and better habits. Salt, caffeine, sugar, and alcohol are all triggers for PMS symptoms, so reducing some, or all, of them will greatly increase your overall well-being.

What Are the Culprits in Your Diet?

If you started your day with a bagel and cream cheese, followed by a tall latte, no sugar; or a cup of cottage cheese, canned peaches, and a glass of orange juice; or even a bowl of instant oatmeal and some tea with milk, you've already had several of the biggest problem foods for women with PMS—and that's just breakfast! The cream cheese, bagel, and oatmeal contain sodium; the latte and tea are high in caffeine; and the peaches and orange juice are high in sugar.

Of course, there is an upside to most of these foods as well: cream cheese, cottage cheese, and milk are dairy products that provide calcium (which can alleviate your PMS symptoms), while peaches and orange juice provide a vitamin boost. Instant oatmeal, while not as healthful as the long-cooking kind, is still a whole grain and contains needed fiber for your diet; and the bagel can be a healthful option if it's whole wheat.

This pro and con snapshot illustrates that making PMS-friendly food choices is not altogether simple. However, it is possible. You just have to be aware of the diet culprits and the diet boosters: Sodium, caffeine, and sugar worsen some PMS symptoms, while dairy or soy can improve them.

Say No to Salt

Sodium is vital to your health. It helps maintain your blood pressure and blood volume, and it's also needed for your muscles and nerves to function properly. But sodium has a potent downside: it carries a number of health risks and it causes bloating—a common complaint of women with PMS.

Your kidneys regulate the level of fluid in your body, causing you to retain water or excrete fluids. When you consume sodium, the kidneys increase the amount of water you retain in order to keep your body's electrolyte balance constant. This is what causes that puffy look associated with bloating. From a health perspective, consuming large amounts of sodium is associated with high blood pressure, a risk factor for stroke, heart disease, heart attack, and kidney failure.

Discerning Between Salt and Sodium

Although you may think of them as the same thing, salt and sodium are not interchangeable. Table salt is one source of sodium, but it's certainly not the only one and it's not even the biggest one. Instead, that honor goes to processed foods, which are the biggest source of sodium in the diet.

Table salt, or sodium chloride, is about 40 percent sodium. Reducing the salt you cook with or use to flavor your foods is a good strategy, especially if you want to reduce bloating. Most foods naturally contain some sodium—for example, milk, beets, celery, even drinking water!

But processed foods, which use salt as a flavor enhancer or preservative, are especially harmful to your diet and are the major cause of bloating, mainly because they contain much higher amounts of sodium than what you might get by seasoning your food at the table with a salt-shaker. However, you should still monitor your salt intake—no matter what foods you consume.

Most Americans consume two to three times the amount of sodium they should—between 4,000 and 6,000 milligrams per day, while the daily recommended value is only 2,000 milligrams. The majority of daily intake of sodium—more than 75 percent—comes from processed foods, while table salt and natural foods account for only 10 percent each.

In addition, look out for these food additives that don't explicitly state they are, or contain, sodium:

- Monosodium glutamate (MSG)
- Baking soda and baking powder
- Disodium alginate
- Sodium benzoate
- Sodium hydroxide
- Sodium nitrate
- Sodium propinate
- Sodium sulfite

 Alert

Just because something doesn't taste salty doesn't mean it's not high in sodium. Many foods, from condiments to ice cream, contain salt as a flavor enhancer or preservative. Here's just a partial list: ketchup, soy sauce, mayonnaise, barbeque sauce, salad dressings, canned soups, canned vegetables, bacon, ham, Ramen noodles, frozen dinners, macaroni and cheese mixes, processed cheeses, bread, dried fruits, tomato sauce, and cake mixes.

A Word about Salt Substitutes

If you can't have salt, you might think, 'Why not a salt substitute?' But salt substitutes contain potassium chloride, which can be dangerous to certain individuals. Too much potassium puts a strain on your kidneys, while too little or too much can cause heart rhythm problems for people with heart disease. Better options are to use herbs and spices, rather than salt, to season your food; to reduce the amount of salt you use while cooking and baking (e.g., using half a teaspoon in recipes that call for one teaspoon of salt), and to avoid salty or processed foods.

 Fact

In 2004, researchers at the National Heart, Lung, and Blood Institute published a study in the *American Journal of Public Health* that concluded that cutting salt levels in restaurants and packaged foods in half would save 150,000 lives.

Cut Back on Caffeine

Caffeine is the world's most popular stimulant. Some 90 percent of adults in North America consume it every day, generally in coffee, tea, chocolate, soft drinks, or energy drinks. For women with PMS, however, caffeine can cause or worsen insomnia and irritability.

Caffeine stimulates the nervous system and is associated with a host of positive effects: it makes you more alert and wakeful, produces clearer and faster thinking, increases your focus, and provides better body coordination. It also improves mental and physical performance. A number of studies over the years have shown that athletes who ingested or received a dose of caffeine had more endurance than those who did not.

Caffeine is also used in combination with medicines to increase their effectiveness. For example, pain relievers are more effective and quick-acting because caffeine helps absorb headache medication.

Alert

Women taking oral contraceptives will experience the effects of caffeine longer than women who are not—a lot longer! Caffeine's half-life—the time it takes your body to eliminate half the caffeine consumed at a particular time—is thirteen hours for women taking oral contraceptives. In contrast, the half-life of caffeine is three to four hours for women who are not taking oral contraceptives.

But too much caffeine can cause irritability, muscle twitching, and even heart palpitations. As few as three or four cups of coffee can cause a condition known as caffeine intoxication, in which a person becomes agitated, nervous or excited, flushed in the face, has a rambling flow of thought and speech, and an irregular or rapid heartbeat.

You can lessen your PMS symptoms by reducing the amount of caffeine in your diet. That means you should cut down or eliminate coffee, tea, chocolate, colas, and energy drinks from your diet, especially in the luteal phase.

Not Too Sweet

Sugar has a host of negative effects on PMS. For one, consuming sugar or sugary foods causes your blood glucose levels to spike and then fall rapidly. This yo-yoing can cause mood swings, headaches, and irritability. Second, consuming too much sugar easily leads to overeating and weight gain: your body feels full when you eat a sugary food, but since sugar is quickly metabolized, you promptly feel hungry again, so you'll probably eat some more. These empty calories add up, as do the pounds, and being overweight is a risk factor for PMS. Third, the more sugary foods in your diet, the less likely there will be room for whole foods. As a result, you miss out on necessary vitamins and nutrients, leading to overall ill health.

L. Essential

> A 1991 study of 853 women, published in the *Journal of Reproductive Medicine*, found that women with premenstrual syndrome were more likely to consume foods and beverages that are high in sugar or taste sweet than women without PMS. The women also ate more chocolate and drank more alcohol if they had PMS.

Experts suspect excess sugar consumption contributes to diseases such as obesity and diabetes, but the evidence is limited. For example, while there is some evidence that consuming too much sugar leads to an increased risk of coronary heart disease, those findings are not definitive. It is clear, however, that consuming too much sugar leads to dental disease and decay.

How Much Is Too Much?

The U.S. Sugar Association, the Institute of Medicine, and the World Health Organization have each weighed in on how much sugar is too much. In 2003, the World Health Organization published a report recommending that sugar (including sugars naturally present in food, added by cooks or consumers, as well as sugars added to foods by manufacturers) comprise only 10 percent of a healthful diet. But a year earlier, in 2002, the Institute of Medicine (a nonprofit organization that advises policymakers, health-care providers, business, and the public) set the upper limit of sugar consumption at 25 percent. Not surprisingly, the U.S. Sugar Association supports the Institute of Medicine report.

High-Fructose Corn Syrup

High-fructose corn syrup (HFCS) is a sweetener made from cornstarch that is added to many foods. It's cheap, tastes sweeter than refined sugar, and blends easily into beverages. In 1966, no one consumed it, but by 2005 Americans consumed 42.2 pounds per year (in contrast, Americans consumed 45.2 pounds of sugar per year).

HFCS is used in all sorts of food products, from soft drinks, fruit juices, and sauces to cereals, peanut butter, potato chips, crackers, yogurt, and meat products, like bacon and hot dogs.

 # Fact

According to the U.S. Department of Agriculture, Americans consume 156 pounds of sugar each year (as of 2003). In 1966, that figure was 113 pounds. Soft drinks are the major source of added sugar in the diet, accounting for 33 percent of total sugar intake. It's not hard to see how that can happen. A sixteen-ounce soft drink alone contains twelve and one-half teaspoons of sugar!

Deciphering Food Labels

By now, many people know that it is important to read food nutrition labels when making food choices. Ingredients are listed by quantity, so if sugar is one of the first few items listed, you know the food is high in sugar. But labels don't always explicitly say sugar; it's known by multiple terms and a food label for a given food often lists several different types of sugars as ingredients.

Alternative names for sugar include dextrose, fructose, lactose, maltodextrins, glucose, glucose polymers, sucrose, invert sugar, raw sugar, honey, cane sugar, turbinado sugar, caramelized sugar, distilled or concentrated fruit sugars, maple sugar, barley malt, date sugar, brown sugar, blackstrap molasses, and of, course, high-fructose corn syrup.

What about Artificial Sweeteners?

Using artificial sweeteners may not be the answer to your diet dreams. A 2004 study in the *International Journal of Obesity* found that artificial sweeteners may interfere with the body's natural ability to count calories based on a food's sweetness.

After feeding two groups of rats either a mix of sugar-sweetened liquid and artificially sweetened liquid, or a sugar-sweetened liquid alone for ten days, researchers offered the rats a high-calorie choco-late snack. Those that were fed the artificially sweetened liquid ate more of their regular food, even after eating the snack. Researchers say the experience of drinking artificially sweetened, low-calorie liquids had damaged the rats' natural ability to compensate for the calories in the snack.

Artificial sweeteners can be almost as confusing as the multiple types of sugar. Here's a primer:

- **Saccharin:** Sweet 'N Low (300 times as sweet as sugar)
- **Aspartame:** NutraSweet, Equal (160–200 times as sweet as sugar)
- **Acesulfame K:** Sunett, Sweet One (200 times as sweet as sugar)
- **Sucralose:** Splenda (500–600 times as sweet as sugar)
- **Neotame:** High-intensity sweetener approved by the FDA in 2002 but not yet widely used in food products (8,000–13,000 times as sweet as sugar)

Drink Less Alcohol

Most experts believe that drinking in moderation is not harmful and may even have health benefits, but for women with PMS, alcohol may do more harm than good.

There's evidence that drinking red wine offers cardiovascular pro-tection, possibly from compounds contained in the grape skins used to make red wine, and there's also evidence that moderate drinking strengthens bones and is associated with a lower risk of developing kidney stones and a lower risk of diabetes.

But alcohol, a depressant, worsens PMS symptoms, especially mood symptoms and can drain your energy level. It may also increase your risk for painful cramping during your period. Ironically, the premenstrual phase may be the time when you are most sensitive to alcohol's effects: progesterone, which drops during the luteal phase, may affect your alcohol tolerance.

There appears to be a mutually negative relationship between alcohol use and PMS: having PMDD (and other affective disorders) is a risk factor for alcohol abuse in women, while alcohol abuse is a risk factor for PMS.

A number of studies have looked at PMS and alcohol; the findings suggest that women with PMS tend to drink more than women without PMS. It may be because the women's PMS symptoms are bad enough that they use alcohol as a coping mechanism, or it may be something else entirely.

What's the Story with Dairy?

Is dairy good or bad for PMS? Most PMS experts encourage women to increase their consumption of dairy products. They are a good source of calcium, which alleviates PMS symptoms; they contain vitamin D, which aids calcium absorption; and they contain the milk sugar, lactose, which also enhances calcium absorption.

Milk and milk products, such as cheese and yogurt are calcium-rich, but not everyone can have them. People who are lactose intolerant, for example, can't readily digest dairy foods. If you are lactose intolerant, consider adding firm cheese, yogurt, and buttermilk, which are all naturally low in lactose, to your diet. Or try lactose-free milk.

Some PMS experts, especially those advocating alternative medicine or vegetarian approaches, believe that dairy worsens PMS symptoms. They argue that the lactose in dairy products can block the body's ability to absorb magnesium, which helps to regulate estrogen levels, and increases its excretion. If you are concerned about getting calcium but want to stay away from dairy, there are plenty of nondairy foods that are rich in calcium, including tofu; green vegetables such as broccoli, Swiss chard, kale, and spinach; okra;

sauerkraut; cabbage; soybeans; rutabaga; figs; salmon; sardines with bones; and dry beans.

Should You Go Soy?

There's some compelling evidence that soy may be a great way to reduce PMS symptoms. Soy products, made from soybeans, contain compounds called isoflavones, which have a chemical structure similar to that of estrogen. A small study in 2005 by researchers at the University of Leeds, England, have found that consuming soy isoflavones reduced the women's PMS symptoms, in particular headache, breast tenderness, cramps, and swelling, as compared to a milk-based placebo.

Soy foods range from vegetables, fiber, and oil, to textured soy protein, such as tofu, soy protein concentrates, and milk and cheese. Here's a brief overview of available soy products:

- Soy fibers
- Soy flour
- Soy protein concentrate
- Soy protein isolates
- Textured soy protein
- Soymilk, made from soaked, ground, and strained soybeans
- Tofu, a cheese-like food made by curdling fresh hot soymilk
- Edamame, also known as soybeans
- Tempeh, a chunky soybean cake
- Soy oil
- Soy nuts
- Soy yogurt
- Soy sauce

Soy fibers, soy protein, textured soy, and tofu can be added to recipes, while soymilk, soy yogurt, and soy butter can replace the dairy versions of these foods.

CHAPTER 17

Great Recipes to Manage PMS

EVEN IF YOU'RE TRYING TO AVOID FOODS that trigger or worsen your PMS symptoms, you still have plenty of options for great tasting and healthful meals, whether they're low salt, calcium rich, low fat, nondairy or caffeine-free.

Low-Sodium Seasoning Alternatives

An easy way to cut sodium is to replace your table salt with other seasonings. You can perk up an otherwise bland meal by adding a variety of herbs, spices, or citrus juices. Here are some healthful alternatives to cooking with salt or adding it at the table:

- Sprinkle vegetables with lemon or lime juice (you can also add finely grated rinds), or try a lemon pepper spice blend to make them more flavorful.
- Opt for black pepper instead of salt on foods like eggs and salads.
- Add fresh salsas that contain lime juice, garlic, onion, and cilantro to corn or asparagus.
- Roast peppers, squash, and other vegetables in some oil, rather than boiling them, to boost flavor.
- Marinate meat, poultry, or fish with onion, garlic, and your favorite herbs.
- Try a French herb mix (it usually contains tarragon, chives, chervil, sage, thyme, rosemary, celery seed, and orange rind) for poultry.

- Add fresh or powdered garlic and fresh or powdered onion, or a salt-free seasoning blend when cooking.
- Mrs. Dash, a salt-free seasoning blend, works for multiple foods, or mix your own.
- Purchase herb or seasoning mixes at specialty spice stores (or their online versions).

Low-Sodium Recipes

Salt may be an acquired taste, but it's very tough to give up once you've acquired it. It can take weeks to adjust to a lower-sodium diet. The following recipes don't taste as though they're skimping on the salt and should make your transition easier.

Orzo with Summer Vegetables

Serves 6

This lovely dish has only 25 mg of sodium per serving.

1 tablespoon unsalted butter
1 tablespoon corn oil
2 medium zucchini, diced
2 medium yellow squash, diced
1 red bell pepper, diced
1 small red onion, diced

Freshly ground black
  pepper, to taste
1 pound orzo, cooked according to package directions,
  without salt, and drained
¼ cup chopped parsley

1. Heat butter and oil in a large skillet over medium heat.
2. Add zucchini, squash, red pepper, and onion. Season with black pepper.
3. Cook, stirring occasionally, for about 12 minutes.
4. Remove the vegetable mixture from heat and combine with cooked orzo in a large bowl.
5. Add the parsley and toss.
6. Serve warm or cool.

Basic Tomato Sauce

Serves 4

**Pasta sauce is a staple for many women with PMS. This is a
fabulous opportunity to make it low salt and reduce bloating!**

2 tablespoons olive oil

1 medium onion, chopped

2 carrots, finely diced

½ teaspoon dried thyme, or 3 to 4 sprigs of fresh thyme

4 cloves garlic, chopped

1 cup red wine

10 fresh basil leaves, chopped

1 bunch parsley, roughly chopped

2 (15-ounce) cans salt-free whole tomatoes,
   or 4 cups chopped fresh tomatoes

Freshly ground black pepper, to taste

1. In a pot large enough for all the ingredients, heat the oil over medium-high heat.
2. Add onion and cook for several minutes, until it turns translucent.
3. Add carrots, thyme, and garlic, and cook for another 6 minutes.
4. Add wine, basil, parsley, and tomatoes, crushing the tomatoes with a wooden spoon or potato masher.
5. Stir well to combine.
6. Season with pepper, and simmer for 1 hour.

Potatoes Rosti

Serves 4

It's so easy to rely on salt when seasoning potatoes, this dish provides a great alternative to your salt shaker. You can serve this for breakfast, or as a nice accompaniment to dinner.

2 pounds (6 medium) potatoes

4 tablespoons unsalted butter

2 teaspoons onion powder

Freshly ground black
  pepper, to taste

Grated low-sodium Gouda
  or Swiss cheese

Sprigs of parsley

1. Peel potatoes and boil or steam them until partially cooked, about 10 minutes.
2. Use the coarse grid of a box grater to grate the potatoes until you have 4 cups.
3. Melt 2 tablespoons of butter, pour the butter over the potatoes, and stir to combine.
4. Stir in onion powder and black pepper.
5. Melt the other two tablespoons of butter in a skillet over moderate heat.
6. Put the potatoes in the skillet and use a spatula to press them flat.
7. Reduce the heat to low and continue to cook for about 20 minutes, until a golden brown crust forms on the bottom.
8. If you think it may be cooking too hard on the bottom (and you're not watching your cholesterol), work a bit more butter in around the sides of the pancake as it cooks.
9. When a nice crust has formed, slide the spatula underneath the pancake to loosen it.
10. Remove the skillet from the heat, and place a large plate upside down over the skillet. Quickly flip the skillet over, holding the plate in place, so the pancake falls out onto the plate, crust-side up.
11. Sprinkle with cheese and a few sprigs of parsley.
12. To serve, cut into wedges.

Stuffed Pork Chops

Serves 4

....

**This entrée relies on low-sodium broth and unsalted butter and
only has 80 milligrams of sodium per serving.**

....

1 tablespoon unsalted butter

1 shallot, minced

10 mushrooms, sliced (use
cremini or porcini, if you
can—otherwise, use super-
market button mushrooms)

Freshly ground black
pepper, to taste

¼ cup low-sodium
chicken broth

¼ cup parsley, chopped

1 teaspoon chopped rosemary

4 thick pork chops

Olive oil

1. Heat a skillet. Add the butter and shallot, and cook for 5 minutes over medium heat.
2. Add mushrooms and black pepper; allow mushrooms to cook down for about 10 minutes, reducing the heat if necessary to prevent burning.
3. Add broth, and deglaze the pan by stirring to dissolve cooked bits of vegetable clinging to the pan.
4. Add parsley and rosemary; turn up the heat, and reduce the liquid until the pan is almost dry.
5. Remove the mushroom mixture to a plate and allow it to cool.
6. Preheat the oven to 350ºF.
7. Wash the pork chops and pat dry.
8. Use a sharp knife to cut sideways into each chop to create a pocket.
9. Fill the pockets with the mushroom mixture.
10. Heat a small amount of olive oil in the skillet and sear the chops on both sides.
11. Transfer the chops to a baking dish, put them in the oven, and bake until cooked through, about 20 to 30 minutes.

Chicken Scaloppini with Mushrooms

Serves 4

2 whole boneless chicken breasts, cut into 4 half breasts

Flour for dredging

2 to 3 tablespoons olive oil

1 cup sliced mushrooms

2 teaspoons lemon juice

Freshly ground black pepper, to taste

½ cup grated low-sodium Gouda or Swiss cheese

Parsley for garnish

1. Dredge a piece of chicken breast in flour; then sprinkle a little more flour on a piece of waxed paper and place the chicken on it.
2. Pound the chicken flat, to a thickness of ¼ inch, using the bottom of a heavy skillet or pot.
3. Repeat with the other pieces of chicken.
4. Heat 2 tablespoons of oil in a large sauté pan, add the mushrooms, and cook over medium heat to the point that they begin to wilt and give up their liquid.
5. Sprinkle with 1 teaspoon of the lemon juice and a grinding of black pepper and stir to combine.
6. Remove the mushrooms and put the chicken pieces in the pan, adding a bit more oil if necessary.
7. Turn up the heat and cook the chicken, just until cooked on the bottom and the edges begin to turn white.
8. Turn the chicken pieces over and place equal portions of the mushrooms on top of each one; then sprinkle generously with grated cheese and with another teaspoon of lemon juice.
9. Turn the heat down to low; cover and cook for a few more minutes until the cheese has melted and the chicken is cooked through.
10. Serve garnished with parsley.

Salmon in a Basil Butter Sauce

Serves 4

Salmon is high in essential fatty acids. This recipe has only 114 milligrams of sodium, so you're doing yourself a favor on both counts!

4 salmon filets, 6 ounces each

1 cup water

Juice of ½ lemon

4 tablespoons unsalted butter

1 shallot, finely diced

1 clove garlic, finely diced

8 basil leaves, roughly chopped

Sprigs of basil for garnish

1. Rinse the fish in cold water and remove any bones.
2. Put the fish in a large sauté pan; add water and lemon juice.
3. Poach the fish in simmering liquid until it has turned pink all the way through, about 8 to 10 minutes.
4. In a small saucepan, combine butter, shallot, and garlic, and cook over low heat only until the butter has melted. Make sure not to brown the butter.
5. Stir in the chopped basil.
6. When the salmon is done, place each fillet on a plate and spoon the butter sauce over and around it.
7. Garnish each fillet with a sprig of basil and serve.

Salade Nicoise

Serves 8

For the Salad:

2½ cups cooked green beans

8 new potatoes, cooked until fork tender and cut into quarters

8 plum tomatoes, quartered

1 small red onion, sliced thin

4 hard-boiled eggs, sliced

2 (6-ounce) cans tuna packed in water without salt

For the Dressing:

¼ cup snipped parsley

1 tablespoon salt-free Dijon mustard

1 teaspoon sugar

¼ cup red wine vinegar

Freshly ground black pepper, to taste

½ cup olive oil

1. Arrange the green beans, potato quarters, and tomatoes on a serving plate with the slices of onion and hard-boiled egg.
2. Drain the tuna and flake it over the top of the vegetables.
3. Whisk together parsley, mustard, sugar, vinegar, and pepper.
4. Drizzle in the oil while continuing to whisk until the dressing emulsifies and starts to look cloudy.
5. Pour over the salad and serve.

Leek and Potato Soup

Serves 8

....

If you want to give the soup a meatier taste, substitute salt-free chicken broth for the water. Avoid using bouillon cubes; they are loaded with sodium!

....

4 leeks, white part only

2 large potatoes

2 tablespoons unsalted butter

3 cups water or low-sodium chicken broth

3 tablespoons chopped parsley

2 to 3 cups whole milk

Freshly ground black pepper, to taste

1. Clean the leeks thoroughly and chop into thin slices.
2. Peel and dice the potatoes.
3. Melt the butter in a large saucepan, add the leeks, and cook for about 10 minutes over moderate heat, stirring to prevent burning.
4. Add 1 cup of water or broth, cover, and cook for a few more minutes.
5. Add potatoes, parsley, and remaining water or broth, and cook until potatoes are tender.
6. Add milk to taste and stir until warmed through.
7. Add freshly ground pepper to taste.
8. If you prefer a creamier soup, transfer the mixture to a blender or food processor before adding the milk and blend until smooth.
9. After blending, return to the saucepan, add milk and pepper, and heat until warmed through.

Flank Steak with Portobello Mushrooms and Wine

Serves 4

Ditch the salt! Sodium contributes to bloating, so if that is one of your primary PMS symptoms (and that's about 95 percent of women), focus on eliminating salt from your diet. Cook low-sodium foods in the premenstrual phase and avoid salt-laden processed foods.

1 flank steak

Freshly ground black
   pepper, to taste

Dash of garlic powder

1 cup red wine

1 shallot, diced

2 Portobello mushroom caps,
   cut into slices ¼ inch thick

1 cup drained salt-free
   canned tomatoes, plus
   ½ cup juice from the can

1 tablespoon dried parsley

Pinch of dried oregano

1. Preheat the oven to 375°F, and place a shallow roasting pan or oven-proof dish inside to heat.
2. Season the steak with pepper and garlic powder.
3. Heat a heavy skillet on top of the stove.
4. Sear the steak in the hot skillet on both sides so that it browns thoroughly and juices are sealed in.
5. Transfer the steak to the pan in the oven to finish cooking (about 10 minutes for medium).
6. Remove it from the oven and set aside.
7. While the steak is cooking in the oven, use half the wine to deglaze the skillet and allow it to cook until almost gone.
8. Add the shallot and reduce heat to low.
9. Add the mushrooms, cook 2 minutes per side, and then remove them from the skillet.
10. Add the rest of the wine and let it cook until almost evaporated.
11. Add the tomato, parsley, and oregano, and simmer for 10 minutes.
12. Return mushrooms to the skillet on the stove, and cook 1 minute to heat through.
13. Slice the steak on the bias, arrange the slices on a plate with the mushrooms and sauce, and serve.

Low-Fat Recipes

Cutting back on fat is one of the healthiest moves you can make, but it can be hard if you're used to eating lots of meat, creamy sauces, baked goods and processed foods. These recipes may just give high-fat foods a run for their money.

Pudge-Free Brownies

Serves 16

No Time to Bake? There are two ways to make great-tasting low-fat brownies—buy a premade mix or make them yourself. Some stores carry the No Pudge! Brownie Mix, which are part of the Weight Watchers diet plan. But if you want a homemade version, try this one.

1 cup sugar
¾ cup flour
½ cup cocoa
2 egg whites (optional, for
   cake-like brownies)
2 teaspoons cornstarch

¼ teaspoon baking soda
¼ teaspoon salt
⅔ cup nonfat vanilla yogurt
   (6-ounce container)
Nonstick cooking spray

1. Preheat oven to 350°F.
2. Mix all dry ingredients.
3. Add yogurt and mix well. Batter will be very thick.
4. Spray an 8-inch square pan with nonstick cooking spray. Spread batter evenly.
5. Bake for 30 to 35 minutes. Remove and cool.
6. Dip a knife in warm water and cut the brownies into 16 squares.

Quick Lasagna

Serves 8

Lasagna is the perfect PMS fix, but a low-fat version is far healthier.

¼ cup grated Parmesan cheese

1 cup part-skim ricotta cheese

1 cup shredded fat-free mozzarella cheese

Nonfat cooking spray

1 (28-ounce) jar spaghetti sauce

1 (12-ounce) package no-cook lasagna noodles

1. Preheat oven to 350°F.
2. In a medium bowl, stir together Parmesan, ricotta, and mozzarella cheeses.
3. Spray a 9-by-13-inch pan with nonfat cooking spray.
4. Spread some sauce on the bottom, and layer noodles atop the sauce.
5. Spread one-third of the cheese mixture over the noodles.
6. Repeat the layers until the ingredients are used up, ending with sauce. Cover with foil.
7. Bake until heated through, about 45 minutes.
8. Remove from the oven, and let cool for 10 minutes before serving.

Low-Fat Pumpkin Pie

Serves 8

This pie has only 240 calories per slice and 7.72 grams of fat.

⅔ cup sugar

⅛ teaspoon salt

½ teaspoon ground cinnamon

½ teaspoon ground ginger

½ teaspoon ground nutmeg

Pinch of ground cloves

1½ cups unsweetened canned pumpkin

1 teaspoon pure vanilla extract

1½ cups evaporated skim milk

½ teaspoon grated orange zest

3 egg whites, lightly beaten

9-inch unbaked pie shell

1. Preheat oven to 450°F.
2. In a bowl, mix sugar, salt, cinnamon, ginger, nutmeg, and cloves.
3. Stir in canned pumpkin.
4. Add vanilla, evaporated milk, orange zest, and egg whites.
5. Beat with an electric mixer until smooth and pour into the pie shell.
6. Bake for 10 minutes.
7. Reduce heat to 325°F and bake until a knife inserted into the filling comes out clean, about 45 minutes.
8. Cool on a rack.

Wonderful Risotto

Serves 2

Parmesan is an intensely flavored cheese, which means that a small amount goes a long way. It can make low-fat foods, such as this creamy risotto, seem indulgent, even when they're not.

2 tablespoons butter
1 medium onion, diced
1 cup medium-grain white
   rice, such as arborio

1¾ cups reduced sodium,
   fat-free chicken broth
½ cup sherry
½ cup grated Parmesan cheese

1. In a large skillet, melt butter over medium heat.
2. Add onion and sauté until golden brown, about 10 minutes.
3. Add the rice and stir until the rice turns yellow.
4. Add the broth and sherry, bring to a boil, and cover.
5. Reduce the heat to low, and cook until the liquid is absorbed and rice is tender, about 20 minutes.
6. Stir in cheese and serve.

Summertime Potato Salad

Serves 8

The low-fat yogurt and flavor herbs and spices in this recipe make the salad very flavorful and healthy.

1 cup plain low-fat yogurt
1 teaspoon ground cumin
1 teaspoon ground coriander
1 teaspoon pepper
2 pounds medium potatoes
   (peeled, boiled until tender, and cut into chunks)

1 large onion, thinly
   sliced into rings
2 tablespoons minced fresh basil
Dash of paprika

1. Make the salad dressing by whisking together yogurt, cumin, coriander, and pepper in a serving bowl.
2. Add potatoes and toss them gently to coat thoroughly.
3. Place onion rings on top, and sprinkle the salad with basil and paprika.
4. Cover and refrigerate for at least 30 minutes.

Calcium-Rich Recipes

You can get more calcium by taking supplements, but you can also get it by eating calcium-rich foods such as green leafy vegetables and dairy products.

Brussels Sprouts in Garlic Butter

Serves 2 to 4

If you've never been a fan of Brussels sprouts, this recipe may change your mind! The Parmesan adds richness, while browning the sprouts adds a slightly nutty flavor.

1½ tablespoons butter

1½ tablespoons olive oil

3 cloves garlic, smashed

15 Brussels sprouts, cut in half

Freshly grated Parmesan cheese (optional)

Salt and pepper to taste

1. Melt the butter and olive oil over medium-high heat until foamy.
2. Reduce the heat to medium and add the garlic. Cook until lightly browned.
3. Remove the garlic and discard.
4. Add the sprouts cut-side down. Cook for 10 to 15 minutes without stirring. The sprouts should be tender when pierced with a knife and browned on the cut side.
5. Top with freshly grated Parmesan cheese and salt and pepper to taste.

Basil Pesto

Serves 4

1½ cups basil

2–5 garlic cloves

¼ cup pine nuts

¼ cup grated Parmesan cheese

⅛ cup lemon juice

⅛ cup olive oil

1. Mix all the ingredients, except the lemon juice and oil, in a food processor.
2. Once everything is mixed, drizzle with lemon and oil.
3. Mix well until blended.

Spinach Parmesan Rice Bake

Serves 8

This great-tasting dish is definitely not low in fat, but it is high in calcium, thanks to the spinach, cheese, butter, and half-and-half. If you want more calcium than you're getting in your supplements and you want to splurge on a meal, this is one to try.

1 package frozen spinach

2 cups cooked white or brown rice

⅓ cup melted butter

2 cups shredded Cheddar or Swiss cheese

¾ cup grated Parmesan cheese, plus ¼ cup for topping

¼ cup chopped onion, or 1–2 large green onions, chopped

1–2 teaspoons fresh minced garlic

3 large eggs, beaten

¾ cup half-and-half (or whole milk)

1 teaspoon cayenne pepper

Salt and black pepper, to taste

1. Set oven to 350ºF.
2. Grease an 11-by-7-inch or 13-by-9-inch baking dish.
3. Cook or microwave frozen spinach, let cool, drain, and squeeze out excess moisture by hand.
4. Combine all ingredients (except the spices and ¼ cup Parmesan) in a large bowl; mix well with a wooden spoon.
5. Season with cayenne pepper, salt, and pepper. Sprinkle with the remaining Parmesan.
6. Bake covered or uncovered for 25 minutes, or until set. Serve.

Soy Recipes

An excellent source of protein, soy can also serve as a dairy replacement for women who are either lactose-intolerant or who want to try it as a way to alleviate their PMS symptoms. These recipes show the diverse ways soy products can be incorporated into your diet—from breakfast to desserts!

Mouthwatering Apple Cinnamon Pancakes

Serves 4

This is a great way to incorporate soy into your breakfast. The vanilla soymilk adds an extra hint of sweetness to these pancakes.

1 cup buttermilk pancake mix

¾ cup vanilla soymilk*

½ tsp cinnamon, ground

⅓ cup apples, peeled and diced, or ⅓ cup apple-pie filling

1. Mix pancake mix, soymilk, and cinnamon until blended.
2. Stir in apples.
3. Cook as directed on the package of pancake mix.

*The amount of soymilk may vary with the pancake mix. Use the same amount of soymilk as the liquid amount stated in the package directions.

Mediterranean-Style Tomato Soup

Serves 18

Mediterranean-style cooking is known for its healthful and flavorful properties. It incorporates a lot of fresh vegetables, uses monounsaturated fats like olive oil, and uses meats, fish, and poultry sparingly. This soup combines the health benefits of a Mediterranean diet with the health properties of soy. One serving provides 11 grams of soy protein and contains only 182 calories.

1 cup chopped onion

2 minced garlic cloves

2 tablespoons vegetable oil

2 quarts vegetable or chicken broth

2 quarts water

3 (10-ounce) cups textured soy protein

2 cups uncooked brown rice

2 teaspoons dried oregano leaves

2 teaspoons dried thyme leaves

1 teaspoon salt

1 teaspoon ground pepper

2 quarts canned diced tomatoes

2 cups diced zucchini

2 cups sliced celery

½ cup chopped parsley (optional)

1. Sauté onion and garlic in oil until tender.
2. Add broth, water, soy protein, brown rice, and seasonings.
3. Bring mixture to boil; reduce heat and simmer, covered, 30 minutes.
4. Add tomatoes, zucchini, and celery; return to boil.
5. Reduce heat and simmer 20 minutes or until rice is tender.
6. Sprinkle with parsley and serve.

Chocolate Monkey Peanut Shake

Serves 2

It can be next to impossible not to give in to your chocolate craving during PMS. But at least this recipe makes up for that indulgence by being low in calories (only 200), nondairy, and low in sodium.

1 cup vanilla soymilk

1 sliced and frozen banana

½ cup ice cubes

2 tablespoons chocolate syrup

1 tablespoon creamy peanut butter

1 teaspoon additional chocolate syrup (optional)

1. Blend all ingredients in a blender on high for 30 seconds or until smooth.
2. Drizzle the optional chocolate syrup in a swirl down the inside of clear glasses.
3. Pour the shake into glasses.

Strawberry Smoothie

Serves 1

Smoothies are a healthful way of being decadent. Try substituting fresh strawberries when they're in season, and garnish with thin banana slices or try soy whipped topping.

1 cup thawed frozen strawberries (including juice)

4 tablespoons water

4 tablespoons soy protein isolate

1 cup crushed ice

1. Mix thawed strawberries, water, and soy protein isolate in a blender.
2. Add crushed ice and blend until smooth.
3. Serve in 12-ounce glasses.

Lemon Tofu Cheesecake

Serves 12

This soy version uses silken tofu, which is softer than regular tofu.
Regular and silken tofu are not interchangeable in recipes.

For the Crumb Crust:

1 cup vanilla wafer crumbs

2 tablespoons finely chopped pecans

2 tablespoons melted soy margarine

1. Combine vanilla wafer crumbs, pecans, and margarine; mix well.
2. Press the mixture into the bottom of a 9-inch springform pan.
3. Bake at 375°F about 8 minutes or until golden brown.
4. Cool on wire rack.

For the Filling:

1½ pounds silken tofu

1 pound low-fat cream cheese

¾ cup granulated sugar

¼ cup all-purpose flour

1 tablespoon grated lemon peel

1 tablespoon vanilla

3 eggs (½ cup)

3 egg whites (⅓ cup)

Chopped pecans (optional)

Thawed frozen berries, as
    needed

1. In mixing bowl, beat tofu until smooth.
2. Add cream cheese, sugar, flour, lemon peel, and vanilla; mix until completely blended.
3. Beat in eggs and whites, one at a time; mix well.
4. Pour filling over crust.
5. Bake at 375°F for 50 to 60 minutes, or until filling is set and edges of top are lightly browned.
6. Cool on wire rack; refrigerate overnight to cool completely.
7. Remove ring and press chopped pecans into sides of cheesecake, if desired.
8. Cut into 12 portions, dipping knife blade in hot water between each slice. Top with berries.

Noncaffeinated Drinks

Reducing caffeine can have a dramatic effect on PMS, but given how ubiquitous it is, it may be hard to give up. If you must have your morning coffee, limit yourself to a single cup, switch to decaf, or try tea, which has about half the caffeine of coffee. If you're looking for alternatives to sodas and energy drinks, and you want something besides water, try iced green tea or seltzer with cranberry juice. Herbal teas also are a good choice, hot or cold.

Italian Cream Soda

Serves 1

Italian cream sodas are a mainstay in some coffee houses and restaurants. They're sweet and rich enough to feel like an indulgence.

8 fluid ounces carbonated water

¾ fluid ounce passion fruit–flavored syrup

¾ fluid ounce watermelon-flavored syrup

1 fluid ounce half-and-half

1. Fill a tall glass halfway with ice. Fill to two-thirds with carbonated water.
2. Pour in the watermelon and passion fruit syrups. (You can also substitute peach or raspberry syrups.)
3. Float the half-and-half on top. Stir when ready to drink.

Sparkling Iced Green Tea with Ginger

Serves 4

This variation of iced green tea is made with a concentrated green tea mixture. To brew it, place three teaspoons for every six to eight ounces of cold water in a sealed container. Let it steep for a minimum of thirty minutes (for a single cup), up to an hour and a half.

1⅓ cups concentrated cold green tea
¼ cup finely chopped crystallized ginger
2⅔ cups ginger ale
Ice cubes

1. Combine concentrated tea and crystallized ginger for at least one hour.
2. Strain and discard the ginger.
3. Pour the concentrated mixture and ginger ale into ice-filled glasses.

Basil Lemonade

Serves 8

This is a light and refreshing drink, perfect for a summer evening. The basil gives it an interesting twist.

1 cup sugar
1 cup fresh basil

1½ cold water
8 cups lemonade

1. In a small saucepan, bring the sugar and water to a simmer over medium heat.
2. Cook without stirring until the sugar dissolves and becomes syrupy, about 5 minutes.
3. Remove from heat, add basil, and let cool to room temperature.
4. Strain the syrup and discard the large pieces of basil.
5. Pour 2 to 3 teaspoons of syrup in an 8-ounce glass; top with ice and lemonade.

Chapter 18

PMS Medications

PMS MEDICATIONS RANGE FROM over-the-counter diuretics such as Midol to antianxiety drugs and selective serotonin reuptake inhibitors (SSRIs). With so many options, it's easy to become overwhelmed or confused. Is it better to take an nonsteroidal anti-inflammatory drug (NSAID), or should you ask your doctor for a prescription for oral contraceptives? This chapter will lead you through all of your medication options.

When Self-Care Isn't Enough

You can reduce stress and eat better, boost your exercise regime, avoid caffeine, and take a dietary supplement, and still be racked with pain! It's not fair, but that's the nature of PMS. With nearly two hundred documented symptoms, and frequently inconsistent symptom patterns from month to month, just when you think you've gotten your PMS under control, the symptoms suddenly shift and leave you miserable.

A Tough Choice

Self-care and lifestyle modifications are the recommended first course of action, but they're not foolproof. The biggest advantage in choosing to modify your lifestyle for PMS-related reasons is that it can be both curative and preventive: a better diet, more exercise, and less stress not only help reduce PMS symptoms but may prevent them from recurring. However, the downside is that the full effects of positive lifestyle changes can take months to develop, and changing your lifestyle is a difficult course of action in general, especially maintaining your new diet or your new commitment to exercise. Lifestyle changes may not relieve all of your physical symptoms either. What do you do in the meantime?

Medications, on the other hand, promise immediate relief, without all of the wait-and-see baggage of lifestyle changes. Or your doctor prescribes a pill that magically eliminates all your symptoms. Except that this doesn't—and probably can't—happen. For one, scientific understanding of PMS is not developed enough for a magic pill, over-the-counter or otherwise. Second, in many cases, medications relieve the symptoms without addressing the underlying causes, like stress, that predispose you to PMS.

When self-care doesn't fully relieve your symptoms, however, medications are a powerful tool in your PMS arsenal. Even women who are adamant about avoiding medications may find themselves backed into a corner when they find their mood swings are out of control or their headaches confine them to bed. Women with mild PMS can treat their symptoms—bloating, achiness, breast tenderness—with some over-the-counter medications. Women with more severe symptoms may find a lot of benefit from taking prescription diuretics, antianxiety medications, or SSRIs, but given their potential side effects, these drugs are not for everyone.

Over-the-Counter Drugs

Over-the-counter drugs for PMS include pain relievers, diuretics, or a combination of both. Companies that sell PMS medications often market several different formulas under the same brand name, with each formula targeting different symptoms, such as cramping, bloating, headaches, breast tenderness. A careful reading of the labels reveals that there are a handful of the same active ingredients in each drug. Over-the-counter PMS pain relievers are used to treat muscle aches, headaches, and menstrual cramps, while diuretics relieve bloating and weight gain. Some also claim to reduce irritability and tension.

Combination Drugs

Midol, made by Bayer Corporation, is one of several over-the-counter drugs that combine pain relievers and diuretics. Its active ingredients are acetaminophen (500 milligrams in each tablet or caplet), the diuretics pamabrom and pyrilamine maleate, and caffeine. There are several different formulations of Midol, each packaged to address a different group of symptoms—for example, cramps and body aches and premenstrual syndrome. The active ingredient in the cramps and body aches formula is ibuprofen; the extended relief formula contains naproxen sodium.

Pamprin, made by Chattem, Inc., is another combination pain reliever/diuretic. Like Midol, Pamprin also comes in several formulations. Its multisymptom formula contains the same active ingredients as Midol, but Pamprin's packaging identifies pyrilamine maleate as an antihistamine rather than a diuretic. Pamprin All-Day formula contains naproxen sodium, while its cramp-relief formulation contains 250 milligrams of acetaminophen, 250 milligrams of magnesium salicylate, another pain reliever, and the diuretic pamabrom.

 Fact

Antihistamines are drugs that block histamine, a chemical released by the body during allergic reactions. They're used to treat allergies and colds and are present in some PMS medications. In PMS medications, the antihistamine is usually included to reduce irritability and tension. Antihistamines have a number of side effects, most notably, sleepiness but also tinnitus (ringing in the ears), dizziness, dry mouth, diarrhea, headaches, and even insomnia.

Premsyn PMS, also manufactured by Chattem, has the same active ingredients as Midol and Pamprin: acetaminophen, pamabrom, and pyrilamine maleate.

Ibuprofen

Ibuprofen, a nonsteroidal anti-inflammatory drug, is one of the most commonly used pain relievers for PMS and menstrual cramps. It's primarily sold under the brand names Advil, Motrin and Nuprin, but also Midol Cramp, and Genpril. Ibuprofen reduces inflammation, fever, and pain by blocking the enzyme that make prostaglandins, chemicals that cause muscle contractions, such as uterine cramping, and pain. Prostaglandins also serve a protective role in the stomach, and because NSAIDs like ibuprofen block prostaglandin synthesis, stomach upset is a common side effect of the drugs.

Low doses of ibuprofen, from 200 to 1,200 milligrams, don't generally cause side effects, but higher doses can cause nausea, diarrhea, upset stomach, high blood pressure, headache, and bloating.

 Fact

> Herbal products that contain feverfew, garlic, ginger, or gingko biloba may interact with ibuprofen and may affect its effectiveness. Talk to your doctor before taking any herbal products to understand how they may affect any other medications you are taking (even over-the-counter drugs such as ibuprofen).

Generic Drugs

There are generic and store-brand versions of over-the-counter PMS drugs available, usually at a lower price. For example, most stores have generic or store-brand versions of ibuprofen or Midol. However, make sure to compare the active ingredients in the brand name medications with their generic or store-brand counterparts so that you know you are getting the same drugs in the same dosages.

Naproxen

Naproxen is another type of NSAID used to reduce pain, inflammation, and fever. Over the counter, it's sold under the brand name

Aleve. It has a higher incidence of upper gastrointestinal tract bleeding, compared to ibuprofen, but studies show its effects also last longer. NSAIDs like ibuprofen and naproxen are gentler on your stomach than aspirin. NSAIDS are most effective when they're taken the week before your period and continued for four days once your period starts; because of their potential for stomach upset and gastrointestinal bleeding, they should always be taken with food.

Aspirin and Other NSAIDS

Aspirin is the oldest and most commonly used NSAID. It's sold under the brand names Bayer, Ecotrin, and Bufferin. It has the same pain-relieving, anti-inflammation, and fever-reducing properties as other, newer NSAIDS, but it also has an anticoagulant, or blood-thinning, effect. For menstruating women, this means aspirin can increase menstrual flow. In contrast, ibuprofen and naproxen may decrease menstrual flow because they have a vasoconstrictive effect (in other words, they narrow the blood vessels).

When Not to Take NSAIDs

Avoid taking NSAIDs for your PMS symptoms if you are trying to get pregnant. A 2006 study found that NSAIDs increased the risk of birth defects, especially if taken during the first trimester. Canadian researchers compared 93 births diagnosed with birth defects in 1,056 women who had filled prescriptions of NSAIDs in the first trimester, with 2,478 births with birth defects in 35,331 women who had not filled prescriptions. The women who took NSAIDs were twice as likely to have babies diagnosed with birth defects, and three times as likely to have babies with structural heart defects. Since it often takes time to suspect and confirm a pregnancy, you can be putting your baby at risk if you take ibuprofen or other NSAIDs in the first few weeks of pregnancy.

Acetaminophen

Acetaminophen, sometimes called paracetamol, is commonly sold as Tylenol. It is a pain reliever and fever reducer, but it does not have anti-inflammatory properties, which means it will not be as effective in reducing symptoms such as breast tenderness, but it will be gentler on your stomach. This makes it a credible choice for women who already have digestive symptoms during PMS.

 Alert

Don't take drugs that contain pyrilamine maleate if you are also taking tranquilizers like Valium or Xanax or sleeping pills. The combination of antihistamines with these drugs could cause extreme sleepiness. Avoid alcohol as well.

Prescription Drugs

Many of the pain relievers and diuretics available over the counter are also available in stronger versions by prescription only. For example, naproxen is sold as Aleve on the shelf in your local pharmacy or grocery store, but is available in prescription strength as Anaprox, Naprosyn, and Naprelan. Similarly, prescription-strength ibuprofen is sold under the Motrin brand name. Other NSAIDs that may be used to treat PMS-related pain include ketoprofen (Actron and Orudis KT if over-the-counter formulations; Orudis and Oruvail by prescription), mefenamic acid (Ponstel), diclofenac sodium (Voltaren), and meclofenamate sodium (Meclomen).

Diuretics

Diuretics eliminate water and sodium from the body by increasing urination. Not only do they reduce bloating, but they also improve mood, breast tenderness, and food cravings. However, because they have potentially serious side effects, diuretics are usually prescribed for women with severe symptoms, rather than for women with mild PMS.

Fact

Diuretics decrease extracellular fluid volume and are used to treat heart failure, liver cirrhosis, hypertension, and some kidney diseases, as well as premenstrual syndrome.

Spironolactone

Spironolactone (Aldactone) is the most commonly prescribed diuretic for women with PMS. It's known as a potassium-sparing drug, which means it does not deplete the body's potassium supply. Spironolactone works by inhibiting the effect of aldosterone, a hormone that affects blood pressure and saline balance. It has a fairly slow onset of action, which means its effectiveness takes several days to develop; conversely, its effect diminishes slowly.

A 1995 study of thirty-five women by researchers at Umea University Hospital in Sweden showed spironolactone significantly reduced irritability, depression, feelings of bloating, breast tenderness, and food cravings over six months, compared to a placebo. A 1991 study of forty-three women showed similar mood improvements over three months.

The standard dose for spironolactone is 50 milligrams per day up to 100 milligrams per day, for seven to ten days during the luteal phase. This intermittent dosing pattern helps minimize side effects, including an increased risk of bleeding from the stomach and duodenum, menstrual irregularities, ataxia (a condition in which a person has problems coordinating muscle movements), drowsiness, and rashes, which are more common during continuous dosing.

You shouldn't take additional potassium if you use spironolactone. In addition, people taking this drug should also avoid salt substitutes.

Hydrochlorothiazide

Unlike spironolactone, which inhibits the effect of the hormone aldosterone, hydrochlorothiazide (Esidrix, Hydrodiuril) inhibits the kidneys' ability to retain water. In addition to PMS-related bloating, hydrochlorothiazide is used to treat high blood pressure and to prevent kidney stones.

Thiazide diuretics cause the body to lose potassium. Eating foods high in potassium, such as bananas and orange juice, is usually enough to compensate for this effect, but in some cases, your doctor may recommend potassium supplements. Hydrochlorothiazide also has a potentially dangerous interaction with calcium. Long-term use of this drug (generally more than six months) can cause calcium to build up in your body and possibly lead to side effects such as calcium deposits.

 Alert

> Thiazide diuretics and licorice don't mix! Licorice root, often taken by women to alleviate chronic fatigue syndrome, fibromyalgia, hypoglycemia, and menopause, can worsen the potassium depletion.

Furosemide

Furosemide is known as a "loop diuretic" because it acts on an area of the kidney known as the loop of Henley that reabsorbs water from urine. Loop diuretics inhibit the reabsorption of sodium, chloride, magnesium, and calcium in the body and increase urine output. The drug, commonly prescribed under the brand name Lasix, is used to treat a variety of serious health conditions, including swelling associated with heart failure, renal impairment, and cirrhosis of the liver. It is also used to treat severe PMS-related bloating, especially if the woman did not respond well to spironolactone.

Fact

Furosemide has been used to prevent thoroughbred race horses from bleeding through the nose during races. It is one of the drugs included on the World Anti-Doping Agency's banned drug list because it is allegedly used as a masking drug.

Oral Contraceptives

Oral contraceptives are only effective against PMS if they contain both estrogen and a progestin. Progestin-only pills or mini-pills, prescribed for women who are breastfeeding, have high blood pressure, or are at risk of blood clots, don't provide any PMS benefit. Obviously, these drugs are appropriate for women who are interested in contraception as well as in PMS-symptom relief.

Several different brands of oral contraceptives are prescribed for PMS, including Ortho-Novum, Loestrin, Mircette, Triphasil, and Yasmin. These drugs are all known as "triphasic" contraceptives; that is, they vary the progestin/estrogen ratios in three phases over the course of the month. This triphasic pattern more naturally mimics a woman's menstrual cycle. In contrast, monophasic pills have the same dose of each hormone in each active pill, while biphasic pills vary the ratio in two phases.

Essential

Oral contraceptives contain one of two different estrogens, ethinyl estradiol or mestranol, and several different types of progestins. Most oral contraceptives contain ethinyl estradiol. For example, Ortho-Novum contains ethinyl estradiol/norethindrone, Loestrin contains ethinyl estradiol/norethindrone, Mircette contains ethinyl estradiol/desogestrel, Triphasil contains ethinyl estradiol/levonorgestrel, and Yasmin contains ethinyl estradiol and drospirenone.

A 2001 study published in the *Journal of Women's Health and Gender-Based Medicine* found that oral contraceptives improved appetite, acne, and food cravings but did not improve mood-related symptoms. The study compared eighty-two women taking either an oral contraceptive or a placebo over three months.

Oral contraceptives also have other benefits beside PMS relief and pregnancy prevention. For example, they can prevent or reduce acne by reducing androgens (male hormones); relieve menstrual pain, prevent some types of ovarian cysts, and protect against the symptoms of fibrocystic breast disease.

 Alert

Drospirenone contains potassium. Yasmin is the only oral contraceptive that contains drospirenone; it should not be taken by women who have kidney, liver, or adrenal disease, take potassium-sparing diuretics (such as spironolactone), potassium supplements, blood thinners, and use NSAIDs over the long-term.

Antidepressants

Antidepressants are the big guns of PMS medications: they are powerful drugs that are effective in reducing mood symptoms for women with severe PMS and PMDD. The two major types of antidepressants are selective serotonin reuptake inhibitors (SSRIs) and tricyclic antidepressants.

SSRIs

SSRIs are the preferred treatment for severe PMS. They alleviate not only PMS-related mood symptoms, but they often help the physical symptoms as well. The main SSRIs used to treat PMS symptoms are fluoxetine, sertraline, and paroxetine.

Common side effects of SSRIs include nervousness, restlessness, nausea, diarrhea, and sexual problems. They may also cause loss of appetite or weight gain.

Another problem is the SSRIs discontinuation syndrome, in which suddenly discontinuing an SSRI can lead to physical and psychological withdrawal symptoms. Women who try an SSRI in response to an emotional crisis and want to stop the drug may find that withdrawal is more difficult than they anticipated.

These drugs are also known to cause sexual dysfunction such as a loss of libido and the inability to orgasm. In 2004, the Center for the Evaluation of Risk to Human Reproduction, part of the National Institutes of Health, released a report that stated that fluoxetine was not only toxic to the fetus of a pregnant women, but that it also had "reproductive toxicity" because of its effect on sexual function. The drug may change the length of the menstrual cycle.

SSRIs take anywhere from a few days to six weeks to be fully effective. There's also a degree of fine-tuning involved: you and your doctor may have to work out the days in which you should take the medication to get the best results. Once you stop taking SSRIs, it takes several days for them to leave your system completely.

Tricyclic Antidepressants

Tricyclic antidepressants were more commonly used before SSRIs were introduced. They work by increasing norepinephrine and serotonin levels in the brain. In contrast, SSRIs let the brain use serotonin more efficiently. Tricyclics also interfere with other neurotransmitter systems and brain cell receptors, causing a variety of side effects, which makes them less desirable depression treatments.

Fluoxetine

In 1988 Eli Lilly introduced fluoxetine in the United States under the brand name Prozac, but when the manufacturer lost a patent dispute in 1991, other drug companies began making the drug. Fluoxetine is used to treat depression, premenstrual dysphoric disorder (PMDD), panic disorder, obsessive-compulsive disorder, and bulimia.

Some doctors also use it to treat attention–deficit hyperactivity disorder (ADHD), anorexia nervosa, and a host of other conditions, although the drug hasn't been officially approved to treat them.

Fluoxetine is has a strong energizing effective, which is why it is such an effective treatment for depression and other mood disorders. Fluoxetine is sold under the brand name Sarafem to treat PMDD. Chapter 11 provides an overview of the controversy surrounding the use of fluoxetine to treat PMDD.

Sertraline

Sold under the brand name Zoloft, sertraline is another SSRI used to treat severe PMS symptoms. A 2002 study, funded by Pfizer, the maker of Zoloft, followed 281 women who received doses of either 50 or 100 milligrams of sertraline or a placebo during the luteal phase for three menstrual cycles. The drug was found to improve PMDD symptoms, quality of life, the ability to function, and social adjustment.

Sertraline may also be associated with lower health-care costs compared to other SSRIs, according to a 2001 presentation by PMDD expert Jean Endicott, Ph.D., at the annual meeting of the American Psychiatric Association.

Paroxetine

Paroxetine is the third SSRI approved for treating PMDD. It's also approved to treat depression, obsessive-compulsive disorder, post-traumatic stress disorder, generalized anxiety disorder, and social anxiety disorder. A 2004 study published in the journal *Psychosomatic Medicine* demonstrated that intermittent dosing of paroxetine relieved PMDD-related mood symptoms.

Paroxetine is sold as Paxil CR (controlled release) and is available in doses from 12.5 to 37.5 milligrams.

Essential

SSRIs are usually prescribed for the luteal phase of a woman's menstrual cycle. This is because women with PMDD are likely to have symptoms only during a part of their cycle, and because they generally respond well to the drugs, it's not necessary for them to take SSRIS continuously. Intermittent dosing also lowers the risk of side effects.

Anxiolytics

Anxiolytics, or antianxiety drugs, are used to treat PMDD if SSRIs don't adequately reduce symptoms, or if the woman suffers primarily from anxiety symptoms as part of PMDD. Antianxiety drugs such as lorazepam, alprazolam, clonazepam, and buspirone are used to treat panic disorder, insomnia associated with anxiety, alcohol withdrawal, and epilepsy, and are given before some surgical and dental procedures as a preanesthetic. Lorazepam is sold under the brand name Ativan; alprazolam is sold as Xanax; clonazepam is known as Klonopin; and buspirone is sold as BuSpar.

Anxiolytics can be physically and psychologically habit–forming, and they have a significant number of side effects, including nausea, headache, nervousness, dizziness, and increased hostility and aggression in some people.

Other PMDD Drugs

The tricyclic antidepressants bupropion, nortriptyline, desipramine, and clomipramine have positive effects on one or more PMDD symptoms, but because they have more side effects than SSRIs, they are second-line drugs, used mainly when SSRIs don't produce adequate relief from symptoms. Tricyclics, or TCAs, are used to treat depression, pain, bulimia nervosa, and irritable bowel syndrome.

Venlafaxine is a newer type of antidepressant that may be an effective rapid treatment for PMDD. It is a dual-action antidepressant, meaning it affects both serotonin and norepinephrine. For this reason, it is called an SNRI, or serotonin-norepinephrine reuptake inhibitor. SNRIs may have fewer effects than earlier dual-action antidepressants and may reduce depression more effectively than SSRIs.

Beta-blockers, which are used to treat high blood pressure, cardiac arrhythmia, and congestive heart failure, also combat the physical symptoms of panic and anxiety. Two beta-blockers, atenolol and propranolol, have been found to have favorable effects on PMDD in preliminary trials.

CHAPTER 19

Complementary and Alternative Treatments

COMPLEMENTARY AND ALTERNATIVE MEDICINE, known as CAM, is a broad and diverse collection of medical disciplines and practices outside standardized medicine. It spans everything from herbal medicine, massage, chiropractic, and Reiki to prayer and healing touch. Women who find they don't respond well to conventional PMS treatments, or those interested in a holistic approach to health care, have a lot of alternative approaches to study. CAM therapies that may provide PMS relief include herbal medicine, reflexology, massage, relaxation therapy, light therapy, chiropractic, acupuncture, and aromatherapy. This chapter covers several—although not all—of the most popular treatments.

When Western Medicine Fails

If you're curious about complementary and alternative medicine, you're not alone. A majority of Americans use some sort of complementary or alternative treatment. According to the National Center for Complementary and Alternative Medicine (NCCAM), half of all people who try CAM do so because they think it would be interesting.

A 2002 study by researchers at Ohio State University found that 62 percent of adults use alternative medicine, including chiropractic, acupuncture, massage therapy, breathing exercises, herbal medicine, and meditation. The data, based on survey responses from 848 people, showed that chiropractic was the most common, while acupuncture was the least common. Similarly, according to information released by NCCAM in 2004, 36 percent of people in the United States used some form of complementary or alternative medicine in 2001. If prayer and megavitamin therapy are included, that figure rises to 62 percent. More women than men use CAM, as do people with higher levels of education.

Types of Complementary Medicine

Complementary medicine is used in conjunction with conventional medicine. Alternative medicine is used in place of conventional treatments. NCCAM developed five categories for CAM practices:

1. Biologically based practices use herbs, special diets, or vitamins (in doses outside those used in conventional medicine).
2. Energy medicines use energy fields, such as magnetic fields or biofields (energy fields that some believe surround and penetrate the human body). These practices include Reiki, magnetic therapy, the Chinese practice of Qigong, light therapy, homeopathy, and therapeutic touch.
3. Manipulative and body-based practices involve manipulation or movement of one or more body parts; they include chiropractic, reflexology, Rolfing, and massage.
4. Mind-body medicine enhances the mind's ability to affect bodily function and symptoms through practices such as meditation and yoga.
5. Whole medical systems are complete systems of theory and practice, such as Chinese medicine, Ayurvedic medicine (from India), naturopathy, and homeopathy.

Herbal Medicines

People turn to herbal medicines when they haven't found relief from more traditional medications, if they come from a culture where herbal medicine is more accepted than in the United States, or if they are drawn to using "natural" rather than manufactured products.

Herbal medicines accounted for 18.9 percent of all CAM therapies in 2001, making it the most common alternative therapy. In 1997, herbal products accounted for $5 billion in out-of-pocket spending, and that number appears to be growing at a rapid rate. Just to put things in perspective: nearly one in four middle-aged women in the United States use herbs such as black cohosh, red clover, chasteberry, and ginseng to treat PMS or menopause symptoms, to aid in breastfeeding, or even to ward off the risk of breast cancer.

But popularity doesn't guarantee effectiveness or even safety. The truth is herbal medicines have a lot of hype, but there is limited evidence to support their often extensive claims. It's only in recent years, as recently as 2004, that clinical trials testing herbal medicine have been funded. Herbal medicines are also poorly regulated. They're sold as dietary supplements, without oversight by the Food and Drug Administration, which means that purchasers can't be sure that they're actually getting what they're paying for; the capsules in a given bottle may or may not contain the stated and effective amount of the active ingredient.

 Fact

Herbal medicine is also known as herbalism or physiotherapy. Herbal medicines are used in homeopathy and naturopathy.

Herbal medicine can be found in various forms: teas, tinctures (a liquid form made by steeping a medicinal plant in alcohol), fluid extracts (stronger than tinctures and made with alcohol or glycerin), solid extracts, herbal poultices (solids mixed with vegetable fats), powdered herbs and tablets, herbal creams and ointments, essential oils, and herbal supplements, which may or not be standardized to contain levels of active ingredients.

PMS Herbal Products

A handful of herbal medicines are typically used to treat PMS, including black cohosh, blue cohosh, wild yam root, chasteberry, and dong quai. These herbal products vary in the symptoms they target and in their effectiveness and safety.

Black Cohosh

Black cohosh (*Actaea racemosa*), an herb native to North America, is primarily used to treat menopausal symptoms and menstrual problems, including sleep problems, mood disturbances, hot flashes, and painful menstrual cramping. There have been at least eight studies of black cohosh, mostly German, involving up to two thousand women, but they've focused on the herb's use as a menopausal treatment rather than as a treatment for premenstrual syndrome.

Experts aren't entirely sure what makes black cohosh work. Initially, the herb was thought to activate estrogen receptors (in other words, it functioned like an estrogen replacement), but more recent studies in 1999 and 2001 showed that although black cohosh does bind with one subtype of estrogen receptors, it doesn't exactly have an estrogen-like effect.

Black cohosh is considered safe, except for women with a personal or family history of breast cancer. One small study suggested black cohosh may promote the spread of breast cancer cells to other tissues in the body. It also has some side effects, especially gastrointestinal discomfort. Other, less frequent side effects include dizziness, headaches, nausea, and vomiting, usually occurring with higher doses.

 Fact

Unlike in the United States, where herbal medicines are classified as dietary supplements, in many European and Asian countries, they are tested and marketed as over-the-counter or prescription drugs. In Germany, black cohosh root is approved and sold as a PMS remedy.

There are many brands of black cohosh on the market, but a German brand, Remifemin, is the most widely used and the most studied. The standard dosage for Remifemin is 80 milligrams (40 milligrams taken twice daily); however, there's evidence that half that dose may be just as effective in reducing menopausal symptoms. It takes between four to eight weeks to become fully effective.

Blue Cohosh

Blue cohosh (*Caulophyllum thalictroides*), not to be confused with black cohosh, is often marketed as a uterine tonic and used to regulate the menstrual cycle, ease menstrual cramping, and treat endometriosis. Blue cohosh contains uterine-contracting substances (Native Americans used it to induce labor), and because it is quite toxic, experts don't recommend it for self-treatment. Alternative names for blue cohosh include yellow ginseng, blue ginseng, blueberry root, papoose root, and squaw root.

Wild Yam Root

Wild yam root (*Dioscorea villosa*) is typically used to treat rheumatism and arthritis-like symptoms, as well as menstrual irregularity, cramps, infertility, menopause, and endometriosis. The Native Americans used wild yam root for birth control. Wild yam's use as a PMS remedy stems from the fact that it contains diosgenin, a natural precursor to progesterone and a substance used to make synthetic steroidal hormones. Diosgenin is thought to help balance progesterone; however, there is no evidence that it actually does so.

Chaste Tree Fruit or Chasteberry

Chaste tree fruit or chasteberry (*Vitus agnus-castus*) is an herb approved as a PMS remedy in Germany. It is thought to inhibit the secretion of prolactin, an inflammatory substance that causes breast pain and tenderness. In fact, there is clinical evidence that supports the use of chasteberry for cyclical breast tenderness and fullness. A number of studies have also shown that chasteberry reduces bloating, constipation, irritability, depressed mood, anger, and headache.

The formulation used in many studies is sold as Femaprin, by Nature's Way. When the fruit extract is used, the standard dose is 20 to 40 milligrams per day, but much higher doses, up to 1,800 milligrams, have also been used.

Dong Quai

Dong quai (*Angelica sinensis*), sometimes called "female ginseng," is a root widely used in Chinese medicine to treat gynecological problems, such as painful menstruation and pelvic pain, recovery from childbirth, fatigue, and mild anemia. It is also used to treat high blood pressure, cardiovascular problems, and headache. Scientific evidence is unclear about its effectiveness as a PMS treatment.

Evening Primrose Oil

Evening primrose oil (*Oenothera biennis L.*) comes from the seeds of the evening primrose plant. It contains an essential fatty acid called gamma-linolenic acid (or GLA), which is thought to be its active ingredient. Some clinical evidence suggests that it offers mild relief for breast tenderness. Many women also use it to relive hot flashes, improve mood, cramping, and night sweats. However, a systemic review of clinical trials comparing evening primrose oil to placebos suggested it had no benefit for PMS symptoms. Potential side effects include seizures (for those with seizure disorders or who take evening primrose oil in combination with anesthetics), occasional headaches, abdominal pain, nausea, and loose stools.

Other Herbal Products

St. John's wort, kava kava, milk thistle, dandelion, and valerian are other herbal medicines sometimes used to treat PMS. Valerian (*Valeriana officinalis*) is used to treat insomnia and other sleep problems. Milk thistle (*Silybum marianum*) and dandelion (*Taraxacum officinale*) are used as diuretics. Kava kava (*Piper methysticum*) reduces anxiety, and St. John's wort (*Hypericum perforatum*) is used to treat mild depression. However, some of these herbal products interact with conventional PMS drugs. For example, St. John's wort may interact with SSRIs and oral contraceptive pills, while kava kava may interact with the antianxiety drug alprazolam, so be sure to tell your doctor you are using them, or talk with your doctor before trying them.

Where to Get Herbal Products

Herbal products have become so popular that you can get them in grocery stores, drugstores, and health-food stores. However, health-food stores and specialty retailers, such as GNC, may have a better selection than your local grocery stores. Frequently, alternative medical practitioners offer products for selection. Unless you've used herbal products before, avoid buying them on the Internet as the sheer selection of different dosages and brands can be confusing.

Your best bets are to purchase herbal products where you can get knowledgeable information, find a good selection, and be reasonably certain that you're getting what you're being promised. Since they are not regulated by the FDA, herbal products frequently do not actually contain the ingredients or dosages that are promised on the label. Consumerlab.com is a company that independently tests herbal products. You can get their reviews of supplements on their Web site, *www.consumerlab.com.*

Acupuncture

Acupuncture is an ancient Chinese technique of inserting thin needles just under the skin into particular points of the body to control pain and other symptoms. The practice is based on the belief that a vital energy, called qi, flows freely in the body. Pain occurs when qi is blocked; acupuncture normalizes the flow of qi.

Acupuncture points are sensitive parts of the body used to bring the body's qi into balance. They run along certain pathways, called channels or meridians, on and in the body. An acupuncturist will diagnose a patient by observing and questioning her, paying special attention to her face and tongue, listening for particular sounds, noticing unusual body odors, feeling the muscles, and asking the "seven inquires": chills and fever; perspiration; appetite, thirst and taste; urination and elimination; pain; sleep; and periods and vaginal discharge. Once the diagnosis is made, the acupuncturist inserts thin stainless steel, silver, or copper needles into the skin. Although treatments vary from person to person, on average, the needles stay in about twenty-five minutes. Most people describe the insertion as painless and even relaxing once all the needles are inserted.

 ## Essential

Traditional Chinese medicine divides the body into twelve meridians or channels, some of which correspond to organs in the body, such as the heart, lung, stomach, large intestine, small intestine, gallbladder, bladder, spleen, liver, and kidney. These meridians run along the hands up to the head, the feet to the chest, and the face down to the feet; they comprise three complete circuits of the body.

Acupuncture as a PMS Treatment

A 2002 Croatian study, published in the *Archives of Gynecology and Obstetrics*, found that acupuncture significantly reduced PMS symptoms such as anxiety, breast pain, insomnia, nausea, gastrointestinal disorders, phobias, headaches, and migraines. When compared to a placebo, acupuncture was 77.8 percent effective, while the placebo was only 5.9 percent effective.

Fact

There are different types of acupuncture, including Japanese, Korean, and classical Chinese. Licensed acupuncturists receive between 2,500 and 4,000 hours of training. Other health-care providers, such as dentists, physicians, and chiropractors, also may practice acupuncture; however, they generally have less training.

Chiropractic and Reflexology

You may think that going to the chiropractor will only help your back, but this treatment may also relieve some PMS-related symptoms.

Chiropractic is a noninvasive approach used to treat specific muscular or skeletal problems, sports and occupational injuries, stress, and illness. Chiropractors focus on the nervous system and use the body's musculoskeletal system (muscles, skeleton, joints, ligaments, tendons, and nerves) to diagnose and treat disorders. Chiropractic treatment can involve spinal manipulation (known as adjustment); soft-tissue techniques, such as massage, heat, ice, and kneading; and ultrasound, electrical muscle stimulation, and exercise. Chiropractors don't prescribe drugs.

 Fact

Chiropractic was founded in 1895 by Daniel David Palmer, who proposed that misaligned vertebrae in the spine caused nerve compression and "disharmony" in the body. Palmer believed health problems could be prevented or treated by adjusting the spine. (Chiropractors use about fifty-five different adjustments in practice.) Today, there are an estimated 70,000 chiropractors in the United States.

Women who suffer from PMS-related pain, headaches, stress, and other symptoms may find chiropractic treatment helpful. There is also a small study that suggests women with PMS may have a higher rate of spine-related problems. The 1999 study, published in the *Journal of Manipulative and Physiological Therapeutics* by Maxwell J. Walsh and Barbara I. Polus, assessed fifty-four women with PMS and thirty women without. They found that the women with PMS had more low-back tenderness, low-back muscle weakness, and neck disability compared to women without PMS.

Reflexology

Reflexology uses pressure applied to certain parts of the ears, feet, and hands to promote relaxation and health in other parts of the body. These body parts are "reflex zones" that correspond to other parts of the body.

Reflexology is based on the notion that a vital energy penetrates every living cell. Pressure applied to the nerve endings in the reflex zones frees up the energy and makes you feel better. One well-known reflexology point is the fleshy part of your hand, between your thumb and forefinger, which corresponds to lymph drainage, bronchia, and back muscles; applying pressure to this spot is believed to reduce headaches.

Conventional medicine does not regularly recommend reflexology, but at least one randomized control trial found limited evidence that reflexology could reduce PMS symptoms. A 1993 study in *Obstetrics and Gynecology* found that a weekly reflexology session conducted over two menstrual cycles (for a total of eight treatments) reduced PMS symptoms by 46 percent compared to a placebo (sham) treatment that relieved symptoms by 19 percent.

Progesterone Creams

Progesterone creams are often touted—especially on the Internet—as PMS treatments, but there is no clinical evidence that progesterone is effective in managing PMS. Studies show it is no more effective than a placebo. In 2001, British researchers conducted a review of ten trials of progesterone therapy and four trials of progestin therapy, a progestin-like substance that is more effective when given orally than natural progesterone. The research team, headed by Katrina Wyatt and Paul Dimmock, found that over ten studies, there was no clinical significant difference between progesterone and placebos, although it did appear to work slightly better on physical symptoms than on mood symptoms. Similarly, progestin appeared to be slightly better at relieving physical symptoms than behavioral symptoms, but the effect was not clinically significant.

The bottom line is, don't count on progesterone creams to relieve your symptoms.

Aromatherapy

If you've ever purchased a scented candle, scented body lotion, or bath oil to help you relax, you may have been practicing a watered-down version of aromatherapy, or literally, therapy using smells. Aromatherapy is more than just using pleasant scents to set a mood; practitioners believe it can improve health.

Aromatherapy uses essential oils with specific properties to target physical symptoms. The essential oils are extracted from flowers, herbs, and trees and are massaged into the skin, inhaled, used with teas, or scented in a room. Aromatherapy is used to relieve pain, reduce tension, and fatigue, as well as care for skin. Since pain, tension, and fatigue are such common PMS symptoms, it's no wonder some women use aromatherapy as a PMS treatment.

While there's little evidence that aromatherapy can alleviate PMS symptoms, there is some research to support that certain essential oils have restorative properties. For example, research at the University of Wolverhampton in the United Kingdom suggests that geranium essential oil reduces anxiety, while other scientific research suggests it has a mild sedative effect. However, conventional medicine generally believes that any therapeutic value from aromatherapy comes from the users' strong beliefs that it works, rather than anything significant in the essential oils themselves. Many times, aromatherapy is used in conjunction with other alternative therapies, such as massage and reflexology.

Essential oils are believed to have different properties:

- **Lavender:** Antispasmodic, antidepressant, anti-inflammatory; antiviral and antibacterial, sedative
- **Chamomile:** Anti-inflammatory, antiallergenic, digestive, relaxant, antidepressant
- **Clary sage:** Anti-inflammatory, antiseptic, sedative

- **Marjoram:** Antispasmodic, anti-inflammatory, antiseptic
- **Rosemary:** Stimulates circulation, pain reliever, decongestant
- **Tea tree:** Antifungal, antiyeast, antibacterial
- **Cypress:** Astringent, stimulates circulation, antiseptic
- **Peppermint:** Digestive, antiseptic, decongestant, stimulant
- **Eucalyptus:** Decongestant, antiviral, antibacterial, stimulant
- **Bergamot:** Antidepressant, antiparasitic, anti-inflammatory
- **Geranium:** Antiseptic, antifungal, anti-inflammatory, diuretic
- **Rose:** Antibacterial, antidepressant, antiseptic, antispasmodic, astringent, diuretic, sedative

PMS Blends

If you want to try aromatherapy to treat PMS, you can massage the oils into your skin (especially the abdomen), inhale them (using a diffuser), or put them in the bath.

PMS recipes generally include clary sage, geranium, and lavender; clary sage, chamomile, and rose; or rosewood, rose, peppermint, and ylang ylang. Put one to four drops of each essential oil in the mixture. For example, one PMS blend might have three drops clary sage, four drops lavender, and three drops geranium.

 Alert

Essential oils are very potent! They can irritate the skin and even cause toxic reactions like liver damage and seizures. Always dilute essential oils with carrier oil, such as olive oil, sweet almond oil, or hazelnut oil.

If you want to create a massage mixture, add the essential oils to a carrier oil such as almond, apricot, grape seed, or jojoba oil (roughly twelve drops to one ounce of oil); in the bath, add eight to ten drops of essential oil and soak for fifteen minutes. If you want to inhale it, put the combined mixture into a diffuser.

CHAPTER 20

PMS and Other Health Issues

ARE YOU SURE YOU HAVE PMS? It isn't the only condition that can make your periods a painful experience. Fibroids, endometriosis, mood disorders, and other conditions can also affect your reproductive health, causing pain and confusion. Also other health issues such as attention-deficit hyperactivity disorder (ADHD), eating disorders, and postpartum depression can have many symptoms that are similar to PMS and can even magnify existing PMS symptoms. This chapter will discuss other health issues that may affect PMS.

Fibroids

Fibroids and PMS are distinct medical conditions, but some women may confuse them because some of their symptoms overlap, including pain, constipation, and pelvic pressure.

Uterine fibroids are benign tumors in the uterus. They're extremely common, affecting as many as 75 percent of women. Since they're usually harmless and often symptom-less, many women don't even know they have them.

Fibroids form from uterine muscle cells, which divide over and over again until they grow into a rubbery mass, nourished by a woman's blood supply. Fibroids can be tiny—about the size of a pea or a plant seed—or big enough to distort the uterus. They usually grow in masses, although it is possible for a single fibroid to grow. Generally, fibroids grow in the muscle wall, but as they get larger they can push into the uterine cavity or outside the uterine wall.

Symptoms

Fibroids are most common in women between the ages of thirty and fifty, and between 20 and 50 percent of women have fibroid-related symptoms, especially abnormal uterine bleeding and pelvic pain. Common symptoms include heavy periods; prolonged periods or bleeding between periods; pelvic pressure or pain; urinary incontinence or frequent urination; constipation; backache; or leg pains. The symptoms also vary depending on the size and location of the fibroids. For example, fibroids that grow into the uterine cavity cause prolonged menstrual bleeding, while those that project outside of the uterus can press on the bladder, causing urinary problems, or on the spinal nerves, causing a backache. In pregnant women, uterine fibroids can increase in size and may cause problems during birth depending on their position in the uterus.

It's not uncommon for women to mistake their fibroids for PMS, and to mistake PMS for fibroids, especially since pain and constipation are symptoms for both, while pelvic pressure may be written off as bloating. Doctors aren't sure why fibroids develop, but genetics, hormones, and other chemicals in the body are thought to play a role.

Hormones and Fibroids

Estrogen and progesterone regulate fibroid growth. Fibroids contain more estrogen receptors than normal uterine muscle cells; they also grow when women are in their reproductive years, when estrogen levels are higher, and then decrease or shrink when women undergo menopause. Experts believe that progesterone facilitates the growth of fibroids, and other hormones and chemicals, including growth hormone and prolactin, play a role as well, although that role is not clearly defined.

Some women may have a genetic predisposition to uterine fibroids. For example, black women are two to five times as likely to develop fibroids as white women, and researchers have identified two genes that are associated with some fibroids.

Fact

Uterine fibroids are also called fibromyomas, leiomyomas, or myoma. If they cause symptoms, they are usually treated with surgery, most commonly with a hysterectomy, depending on the woman's desire to bear children in the future.

Diagnosing Fibroids

Doctors generally diagnose fibroids if they feel them during a regular pelvic exam. They may also diagnose them (or confirm their diagnosis) using ultrasound, known as an SIS, which uses fluid to distend the uterine cavity). Physicians may also discover fibroids using a hysteroscopy but only if the woman is having the procedure done for another reason.

Ultrasound uses sound waves to get an image of internal organs. Vaginal ultrasounds are used to look at the pelvic structure and to find small fibroids, while abdominal ultrasounds are used to find large fibroids. Your doctor may perform one or both types of ultrasounds. Sometimes advanced imaging tools such as magnetic resonance imaging (MRI) or computerized tomography (CT) scans are used to confirm a diagnosis.

A hysteroscopy involves using a small telescope to look inside your uterus; sometimes a small sample, or biopsy, is taken of uterine tissue. This slightly painful procedure is done using a local anesthetic, usually in the hospital. This method is especially useful for examining the type of fibroids commonly associated with abnormal uterine bleeding.

Treating Fibroids

Some alternative medicine practitioners advocate progesterone cream as a treatment for PMS and fibroids, based on the notion that fibroids are caused by "estrogen dominance" and the progesterone creams rebalance a woman's hormones. Progesterone creams, they claim, dramatically shrink fibroids.

Conventional medicine treats fibroids with surgery, drugs, and ultrasound treatment. Surgery can mean hysterectomy (a complete removal of the uterus), myomectomy (removal of individual fibroids), or uterine artery embolization (injection of small particles into the blood vessels to cut blood flow to the fibroid and cause them to shrink). For years, doctors recommended hysterectomies as a first-line treatment; in fact, fibroids are the main reason women receive this surgical procedure, accounting for about two hundred thousand procedures annually, or one-third of all hysterectomies performed each year.

In recent years, however, other fibroid-removal techniques have been developed and approved, including a device that uses magnetic resonance image (MRI)–guided ultrasound to target and destroy fibroids. This noninvasive procedure, approved by the FDA in 2004, offers an alternative to surgery. Although this treatment spares a woman's uterus, it's not intended for women who want to become pregnant.

Medical treatment for fibroids uses drugs called GnRH agonists to stop the menstrual cycles. GnRH agonists reduce the tumors and stop bleeding, but they also cause osteoporosis if used over a longer period. In addition, once the drugs are stopped, the fibroids quickly grow again. For this reason, GnRH agonists are usually given for one to three months as preparation for a surgical procedure.

Endometriosis

Endometriosis is a condition in which endometrial tissue, which normally lines the uterus, invades locations outside the uterus, including the ovaries, fallopian tubes, and the abdominal cavity. Since endometrial tissue, regardless of location, responds to a woman's menstrual cycle, tissue that adheres to other organs builds up, breaks down, and bleeds during the course of a menstrual cycle. However, unlike tissue in the uterus, endometrial tissue in other locations is not expelled from the body, instead it pools and causes adhesions, leading to scarring, heavy bleeding, and pain. Endometriosis is the most common cause of secondary dysmenorrhea, in which uterine pain is caused by a medical condition. It is also a cause of infertility problems.

Endometriosis can also cause a feeling of fullness, painful bowel movements during the period, and gastrointestinal problems such as diarrhea, constipation, and nausea. These symptoms lead some women to think they have PMS when they actually have endometriosis.

 ## Fact

More than 5.5 million women and girls in North America suffer from endometriosis. On average, women are diagnosed in their late twenties, although many suffer for years before being diagnosed.

Causes

There are several theories about the cause of endometriosis, although none have been proven.

- Reflux menstruation, in which menstrual tissue backs up through the fallopian tubes and implants in the abdomen
- Distribution by the lymph or blood system, in which endometrial tissue is distributed from the uterus to other parts of the body
- Surgical transplantation, in which tissue is accidentally implanted in the abdominal cavity through surgery
- Ability of the cells in the pelvic region to change into endometrial cells

Reflux menstruation is the most popular theory, but some experts argue there must be another mechanism involved since 90 percent of women experience tissue backup and only 5 percent develop endometriosis. These experts believe immune system or hormonal problems cause the tissue to grow.

Treatments

Many of the same strategies used to treat PMS are used to treat endometriosis. Doctors recommend NSAIDs and oral contraceptives to treat pain and reduce ovulation; other treatments include Lupron, a GnRH agonist which induces menopause-like effects. Surgical options include laparoscopic surgery, a minimally invasive procedure to remove endometrial tissue from the affected organs, and hysterectomy.

 Fact

When endometrial tissue invades the ovaries, it forms cysts known as endometriomas. These cysts are also known as "chocolate cysts" because they are filled with dark blood that resembles thick chocolate syrup.

Psychological Issues

There's a murky and complicated relationship between PMS and other mood disorders. PMS includes as number of mood symptoms, and some mood disorders are subject to menstrual magnification, growing more intense during the premenstrual phase and making it easy to become confused about what's really causing depression, anxiety, irritability, and mood swings.

Lifestyle and personal issues also can masquerade as PMS. Women who are under a lot of stress or who have problems communicating with others and become irritable and angry as a result may write off their feelings and reaction as a PMS rant. Similarly, women who have a history of physical or sexual abuse, or who have substance abuse problems, may deny or dismiss their problems and instead blame PMS for their emotional turmoil.

In addition, these issues are likely to exacerbate existing PMS symptoms, in effect serving as both a foil and an intensifier for PMS.

Attention-Deficit Hyperactivity Disorder (ADHD)

Attention-deficit hyperactivity disorder is often considered a condition that affects children, especially boys. But the neurological disorder also affects adults. Experts estimate that at least 4 million women have adult ADHD, although many of them may be undiagnosed. PMS can aggravate ADHD symptoms, worsening mood swings and making the person more irritable, anxious, and distracted than usual.

ADHD symptoms include the following:

- Hyperactivity, such as fidgeting, feeling restless, and excessive speech
- Forgetfulness
- Poor impulse control
- Distractibility
- Appearing not to listen when addressed
- Avoiding tasks that require concentration and organization
- Mood swings

Experts aren't sure what causes ADHD, but environment, diet, and genetic predisposition are all implicated. Some research suggests that ADHD is triggered by genes that cause a dopamine deficiency. Dopamine is a neurotransmitter that regulates emotion, motivation, insulin regulation, physical energy, and fine-motor coordination.

Other studies suggest dietary factors, such as a lack of omega-6 fatty acids, trigger the disorder. Finally, other possible causes include nicotine (pregnant women who smoke have a higher risk of having children with ADHD), alcohol, lead poisoning, and even some head injuries.

Fact

Attention-deficit hyperactivity disorder affects boys more frequently than girls. About 2.5 boys have ADHD for every girl with the disorder. About 60 percent of children diagnosed with ADHD carry the disorder into adulthood.

Women with ADHD often find that the hormonal fluctuations during their menstrual cycles, perimenopause, and postpartum make their symptoms significantly worse, as can a menstrually induced iron deficiency. In addition, personal issues like physical and emotional abuse, substance abuse, and stress may worsen ADHD symptoms.

ADHD Treatments

Doctors generally treat ADHD with medications that stimulate the areas in the brain responsible for focus and concentration, including methylphenidate (sold under the brand names Ritalin and Concerta), amphetamines (Adderall) and dextroamphetamines (Dexedrine). Other drugs include the antidepressant bupropion (Wellbutrin) and atomoxetine (Strattera), a type of drug known as a norepinephrine reuptake inhibitor.

Women with PMS and ADHD may also benefit from counseling and coaching, in which they learn about the stressors that worsen their PMS and how to ameliorate their ADHD symptoms by learning how to organize, prioritize, and develop life skills.

Eating Disorders

Severe PMS and eating disorders are related, research shows. A 1997 Italian study of twelve women with PMDD and ten women with either bulimia or binge-eating disorder found that 16.6 percent women with PMDD also had an eating disorder. Eating disorders often exacerbate the symptoms of PMS and PMDD and may cause some of the symptoms associated with PMDD, such as depression.

Women with eating disorders such as anorexia nervosa, bulimia, and binge-eating disorder are also very likely to be depressed; more than 50 percent of people diagnosed with an eating disorder are also diagnosed with severe depression.

Question

What is binge-eating disorder?

Binge-eating disorder is characterized by frequent episodes of uncontrollable eating of large amounts of food. Binge eaters eat rapidly; they eat until they're uncomfortably full; they eat alone because they're embarrassed by the amount of food they're eating; and they feel guilty, disgusted, or depressed after overeating. Unlike bulimics, binge eaters do not purge after eating. Up to 2 million people are affected by the disorder.

Causes

Eating disorders have a mix of psychological and genetic causes. Anorexics, bulimics, and binge eaters often feel out of control and use food as a way to gain control over their lives. Many women with these disorders have deep psychological problems, such as past sexual abuse or violence, and use eating behaviors to avoid confronting these issues. They also tend to be perfectionists with unrealistic expectations of themselves.

Research shows that the brain chemistry of women with eating disorders is altered. A 2005 study in the *Journal of Biological Psychiatry* suggests that anorexics have excess activity in the brain's dopamine receptors. In fact, the disorders themselves encourage changes in brain chemistry: As women undereat and overeat, they activate brain chemicals that produce feelings of well-being and euphoria.

The longer a woman has an eating disorder, the more her brain chemistry is altered and the more difficult the condition is to treat.

 ## Fact

Eating disorders are also associated with a number of other psychiatric illnesses, including anxiety disorders (social anxiety disorder, panic attacks, generalized anxiety disorder), personality disorders, obsessive-compulsive disorder, and depression.

Other causes include a person's personality type, which makes some women more vulnerable to eating disorders; stress, which causes some women to self-medicate with comfort foods and produces hormones that encourage the formation of fat cells; age (young women often don't have the ability to manage emotional impulses); family; and social pressure.

Risk Factors

What puts you at risk for developing an eating disorder? According to the 2004 International Conference on Eating Disorders in Orlando, Florida, risk factors include:

- High weight concerns before age fourteen
- High level of perceived stress
- Behavior problems before age fourteen
- History of dieting
- Mother diets and is concerned about appearance
- Siblings diet and are concerned about appearance
- Peers diet and are concerned about appearance
- Negative self-evaluation
- Perfectionism
- Shy and/or anxious

- Competitive with siblings' shape and/or appearance
- Distressed by life events occurring in the year before the illness develops
- Critical comments from family members about weight, shape, and eating
- Teasing about weight, shape, and appearance

Treatments

Medication and therapy are used to treat eating disorders, but the exact strategy depends on the type of disorder. For example, bulimia is treated with the SSRI fluoxetine (Prozac), but SSRIs and other antidepressants are not effective treatments for anorexia, which is often treated with psychotherapy. Binge-eating disorder may be treated with cognitive-behavioral therapy, psychotherapy, or antidepressants.

PMS and Postpartum Depression

Postpartum depression, or PPD, is depression that occurs in women after they give birth. It can last a few weeks or several months, but the symptoms are similar to major depression that is not related to pregnancy: a loss of interest or pleasure in life, fatigue, loss of appetite, feelings of worthlessness, unexplained weight loss or gain, insomnia, and thoughts about harming yourself, among others. Women with PPD may also have thoughts about harming their baby.

PPD is not the more common and familiar "baby blues" that also occur after a woman gives birth. This condition affects up to 80 percent of new mothers, features rapid mood shifts and includes symptoms such as irritability, crying, problems concentrating, and insomnia. It resolves shortly after childbirth, anywhere from within a few hours to within several days. In contrast, women with PPD have significant symptoms that occur within the first four weeks after childbirth.

PMS and PPD are intimately connected: PMS is a risk factor for PDD, and PPD is a risk factor for PMS. While experts know some of the mechanisms behind PMS, the same can't be said for PPD. Experts do know that a woman's hormones exhibit extreme fluctuations right after childbirth, but studies show that those fluctuations don't appear to cause PPD. In addition, according to researchers, new fathers, who don't experience hormonal fluctuations, can also suffer from PPD. A 2005 study published in the British journal the *Lancet* analyzed data from the Avon Longitudinal Study of Parents and Children and found that 4 percent of fathers (compared to 10 percent of mothers) reported feelings of anxiety, hopelessness, and irritability within eight weeks of their child's birth.

Social factors, on the other hand, appear to play a role. Stress, poor marital relationships, previous depression, and a lack of support systems, all risk factors for PMS, are also correlated with whether a woman gets PPD. Other factors may include the dramatic lifestyle changes after having children, being a single mother, having an unwanted or unplanned pregnancy, and having an infant with temperament problems, such as colic.

Women who have PPD with one pregnancy are also more likely to experience it in subsequent pregnancies.

Postpartum Psychosis

Postpartum psychosis is an extreme form of PPD in which a woman experiences a complete break with reality. PPP is rare: only 1 in 500 to 1 in 1,000 women experience it in the first delivery. (The risk dramatically rises to one in three for women who've had it in previous pregnancies.) Many women with PPP aren't even aware that they have the condition. The most famous example of a woman with PPD in recent years is Andrea Yates, a Texas mother who drowned her five children. This mental illness is treated with antipsychotic medications.

Ⅼ. Essential

Experts have studied whether consuming omega-3 fatty acids can help alleviate symptoms of major depressive disorders such as PMDD and PPD. Studies have shown, for example, that woman who consume more fish and seafood, which contain these fatty acids, are less likely to suffer from PPD. Fish consumption, in general, is associated with lower rates of depression and fewer thoughts of suicide.

Menstrual Magnification

PMS also worsens a number of other conditions, from allergies to sea-sickness, and is associated with smoking and alcohol consumption. In fact a number of chronic disorders worsen during PMS, including the following:

- Epilepsy
- Multiple sclerosis
- Systemic lupus erythematosus
- Inflammatory bowel disease
- Irritable bowel syndrome
- Diabetes
- Asthma

Up to 40 percent of women with asthma find it gets worse during PMS. Experts think this is because PMS makes women more vulnerable to stress, which in turn intensifies the effects of asthma, lowers a woman's resistance to infection, and increases the hyper-reactivity of the airways in her lungs.

Diabetes also worsens during PMS. High levels of estrogen and progesterone affect insulin. A study of women with insulin-dependent diabetes showed that 27 percent experienced higher blood sugar levels in the week before their menstrual period than at other times in their cycles, while 12 percent experienced lower levels in that week before their periods. However, some experts say these changes are the result of cravings and dietary responses to PMS, not to insulin changes.

CHAPTER 21

The End of PMS?

PMS IS NO PICNIC, but neither are perimenopause and menopause. Women in their forties, fifties, and beyond suffer from hot flashes, night sweats, decreased libido, and a host of other symptoms. This chapter will help you learn what you can do to make the transition smoother and less disruptive.

The PMS Life Cycle

PMS ends when women undergo menopause. It's often a difficult transition; PMS-related breast tenderness and bloating give way to menopause-related hot flashes, night sweats, and vaginal dryness, as well as health conditions like osteoporosis. For women who spent years suffering from PMS or PMDD, however, this shift can be a dramatic relief.

Treatment of PMS, PMDD, perimenopause, and menopause is critical. Without it, if you have PMS as a young adult, you can potentially suffer from symptoms associated with your menstrual cycle for decades!

 Fact

Osteoporosis is a condition in which bones become very porous and break easily. Menopausal women are at high risk for developing this disease. You can prevent osteoporosis by quitting smoking, exercising regularly, limiting alcohol, and consuming a diet that provides adequate calcium and vitamin D.

While PMS can affect women of any age, it seems to peak when women are in their thirties. Since premenstrual syndrome is so often hard to diagnose, women may struggle for years before they recognize, understand, and can treat their condition.

About a decade later, those same women start perimenopause. During this phase, they begin to experience some symptoms associated with menopause, such as hot flashes, as well as their usual PMS. By their fifties, most women have moved on to full-blown menopause, along with its array of health effects and severe symptoms. Given this scenario, doesn't it make sense to alleviate your PMS symptoms now rather than trying to wait it out in the hope that things will get better on their own?

Perimenopause

Have your periods started to fluctuate? Do you occasionally have hot flashes, problems sleeping, or a decreased libido? If you're in your thirties or forties, you may be in perimenopause, the transitional phase that precedes menopause.

It can be hard to tell when you're actually in perimenopause since it doesn't have a specific starting point, such as a particular age, and its end point is defined in relation to menopause. In other words, perimenopause is over only after you've entered menopause. Moreover, if you've had PMS symptoms for years, it may be even more difficult for you to realize that your PMS symptoms are now part of perimenopause.

In general, perimenopause (which literally means "around menopause") takes place when a woman is in her mid-forties. However, this transitional phase can start as much as a decade earlier, when a woman is thirty-five—a time of prime adulthood, when most people consider themselves too young to be aging. Perimenopause also varies in length: it can last as little as a year or as long as six years, or even up to a decade.

The Process

So what happens during this time? As you age, your body's reproductive system gradually slows and, for a time, goes a bit haywire: your ovaries begin to produce less estrogen and progesterone, your hormone levels start to fluctuate wildly, your periods become irregular, sometimes bunching up and other times disappearing for a couple of cycles, and your fertility decreases. This is why older women generally have a more difficult time getting pregnant.

 Alert

Motherhood delays perimenopause! Childless women are more likely to enter perimenopause sooner than women with children. The more children you have, the later you are likely to experience the onset of perimenopause.

Symptoms

Perimenopause is transitional in nature, and its symptoms resemble the symptoms of both menopause and PMS. They include irregular periods, mood changes, headaches, difficulty concentrating and forgetfulness, joint and muscle aches, difficulty sleeping, changes in sexual desire, night sweats, hot flashes, vaginal dryness, extreme sweating, and frequent urination and urinary incontinence.

Irregular periods are the most common perimenopausal symptoms, affecting nine out of ten women, while 85 percent report hot flashes and sleep problems. During a hot flash, you'll suddenly feel your face, neck, chest, arms, and back get intensely hot, and your skin becomes flushed and blotchy. The sensation lasts only between three to five minutes, but it can take as long as thirty minutes to recover, and you may also experience sweating, chills, and shivering as your body temperature readjusts.

In some women, perimenopause kicks off more intense PMS symptoms.

Hormonal Changes

Perimenopausal symptoms are mostly caused by changes in hormone levels, which don't simply decline during perimenopause, but rather rise and fall wildly, peaking, then dropping abruptly, and rising again. This is caused by the aging of the ovaries, which, after decades of regular hormonal cycles, produce less estrogen and progesterone in perimenopause. In response, the pituitary gland compensates by increasing the amount of follicle-stimulating hormone (FSH) and luteinizing hormone (LH) it secretes to stimulate follicles. The maturing follicles raise estrogen and progesterone levels again: they first produce estrogen, and then, after ovulation, progesterone. However, this is a short-term solution; over time, the pituitary gland has to produce more and more FSH and LH to keep the process going, until at last, estrogen and progesterone ultimately decline and you enter menopause. Women in menopause have high levels of FSH.

Compared with younger women, women in perimenopause:

- Have higher amounts of follicle-stimulating hormone (FSH levels start to rise about five years before menopause)
- Have higher levels of luteinizing hormone (which starts to rise about one year before menopause)
- Have occasional high levels of estriadol (one type of estrogen), as FSH stimulates follicles
- Have gradually decreasing levels of estrogen and progesterone

Where Does Estrogen Fit In?

Research shows that estrogen levels can intensify the body's response to stress. In a 2004 study, Yale researcher Rebecca M. Shansky and her colleagues subjected rats to mild stress and then gave them a short memory test. Without stress, both male and female rats performed well on the tests and performed equally well after experiencing higher levels of stress. However, mild stress affected the female rats more. Shansky found that the responses were associated with the animals' high estrogen phase and concluded that high levels of estrogen enhance the body's stress response and cause greater stress-related cognitive impairment.

 ## Fact

> Ovarian function starts to change around age thirty-eight. This is one reason older women are more likely to have twins. A 2006 Dutch study published in the journal *Human Reproduction* found that women in their thirites, especially thirty-five and older, have higher levels of follicle-stimulating hormone and were more likely to prepare more than one egg per menstrual cycle.

What does this have to do with perimenopausal women? Plenty, some experts believe.

For one, while perimenopause is usually described as a time when estrogen decreases, some studies have found that estrogen levels are actually higher in perimenopausal women than in younger women. Second, perimenopausal women don't ovulate every menstrual cycle. This means that for perimenopausal women, estrogen levels increase in the first half of their menstrual cycle, but because they don't ovulate, the pituitary gland secretes FSH to stimulate another follicle, which makes high estrogen levels rise again about a week or so later. This peak in estrogen not only induces physical premenstrual symptoms like breast tenderness (especially in the front of the breast) and stretchy cervical mucus (which increases as estrogen levels rise and is associated with ovulation), but also induces stress-related symptoms.

Jerilynn C. Prior, M.D., a Canadian endocrinologist and director of the Center for Menstrual Cycle and Ovulation Research, argues that high estrogen levels coupled with intermittent ovulation (which is common in older women whose reproductive function is declining) explains why perimenopausal women have symptoms such as hot flashes and night sweats, changes in libido, and PMS symptoms.

Fact

Declining estrogen can cause urinary incontinence in perimeno-pausal and menopausal women. Estrogen loss weakens the muscles around the urethra, leading some women to leak urine when they cough, laugh, or sneeze.

Depression and Perimenopause

Depression accelerates perimenopause. A 2003 study in the jour-nal *Archives of General Psychiatry* found that women with depression begin perimenopause earlier than women who are not depressed. Researchers followed 1,000 women ages thirty-six to forty-six for three years and found that those with a history of depression were more likely to display symptoms such as changes in their menstrual cycles and missing periods, or they had to begin hormone replace-ment therapy earlier to regulate their cycles and alleviate symptoms such as hot flashes and flushing. Experts speculate that depression may slow the production of hormones.

Poor women are also more likely to go through perimenopause and menopause earlier, research shows. A 2003 study published in the *Journal of Epidemiology and Community Health* found that women who experience lengthy periods of economic hardship became peri-menopausal sooner. Study author Lauren Wise speculates that stress, poor nutrition, or toxins such as lead and tobacco accelerate egg depletion, which is known to trigger perimenopause.

Are You Experiencing Perimenopause?

If you want to learn if you're in perimenopause, you may be tempted to buy an over-the-counter test that promises to tell you. However, these tests measure levels of FSH, which rise and fall over the course of the menstrual cycle, even in aging women. So while the test may be able to tell you that your FSH is elevated, it can't tell you that you're definitively in perimenopause.

Researchers have actually found that a woman's own self-assessment, not a separate "objective" test, was the most accurate way to determine perimenopause. In 2003, investigators from Duke University reviewed research from 1966 through 2001 and found that there was no one symptom or test to confirm or rule out perimenopause. The most accurate ways of determining this phase were, in descending order: a woman's own self-assessment, hot flashes, night sweats, vaginal dryness, high follicle-stimulating hormone levels, and low inhibin B levels (a chemical that suppresses FSH).

 Alert

Don't assume perimenopause means you can't get pregnant! Irregular cycles and irregular ovulation may indicate declining fertility, but perimenopausal women can still get pregnant.

Perimenopause Treatments

Some treatments for perimenopause are similar to PMS treatments, while others are used to treat more menopause-like symptoms. They include the following:

- Low-dose oral contraceptives, which help regulate periods and may reduce hot flashes and sleep problems, as well as prevent unwanted pregnancy
- Antidepressants to help stabilize moods
- Progestin (sometimes called the minipill) to reduce irregular bleeding and for nursing mothers
- Estrogen creams, applied topically around the vaginal area, to reduce dryness

Lifestyle changes can also reduce symptoms and prevent health problems related to menopause:

- Exercise, especially strengthening exercises, help prevent muscle loss, while stretching exercises help you stay flexible.
- Add soy to your diet to reduce hot flashes and other symptoms. Soy contains isoflavones, which have estrogen-like properties.
- Calcium supplements help prevent bone loss.
- Alternative therapies such as yoga may help relieve emotional symptoms by reducing stress, as well as provide health benefits, such as increased fitness.
- Some herbal treatments such as evening primrose oil, black cohosh, and ginkgo biloba may be effective in relieving symptoms such as hot flashes, mood swings, and night sweats. But always use herbal products with caution and consult your physician before taking them.

Menopause

Menopause occurs when you stop having menstrual periods for twelve months. It is the culmination of the transitional perimenopause phase when your body's reproductive system slows down. By menopause, the ovaries stop producing estrogen, which leads to myriad symptoms including hot flashes (sometimes followed by intense cold, shivering, and sweating), night sweats, sleep problems, urinary problems, vaginal dryness, osteoporosis, joint and muscle pain, back pain, skin changes (less elasticity, thinning, and wrinkling), breast atrophy, forgetfulness, irritability, fatigue, and a loss of sexual interest.

On average, women experience the onset of menopause at fifty-one, but it varies depending on the woman. However, it generally happens between forty and fifty-eight. About 1 percent of women will experience premature menopause, which is defined as menopause that occurs before age forty, and each year, about 263,000 enter surgical menopause after having their ovaries removed.

Alert

> Autoimmune disorders, such as lupus or Crohn's disease, thyroid disease, and diabetes can all cause premature menopause.

Menopause can be devastating for some women, not only because of the associated physical symptoms, but because it marks the end of their fertility, which they experience as a loss of womanhood. On a biological level, the estrogen loss associated with menopause may increase a woman's risk of depression. A Dutch study published in the journal *Mauritas*, found increased rates of depression as women began to experience perimenopause, and as they transitioned from perimenopause to menopause.

 Fact

> According to the North American Menopause Society, the average age of menopause hasn't changed for several centuries, despite longer life expectancy.

Physical Changes

In addition to the typical symptoms brought on by hormonal changes, menopausal women experience a number of physical changes: the skin is less elastic, thinner, and prone to wrinkling; the metabolism slows down, which causes weight gain (especially around the waist); become more forgetful; at higher risk for osteoporosis, which makes bones brittle and prone to breakage, and may even cause "shrinking" in height and affect posture; and a higher risk of heart disease.

Researchers have found that a drop in estrogen and progesterone can increase appetite. Investigators at Oregon Health and Science University, Portland, studied the hunger levels of monkeys that had their ovaries removed and found that in the absence of ovarian hormones, the monkeys increased their food intake by 67 percent and gained 5 percent body weight in a matter of weeks.

Menopause Tests

Just as for perimenopause, the best way to tell if you're in menopause is to gauge your own symptoms. However, if you're concerned that you may be entering menopause prematurely and want to you ask your doctor for tests, here is what you can expect.

Tests for premature menopause may include an FSH blood level measurement, which measures the level of follicle-stimulating hormone and is used to test fertility. The test is usually taken on day three of the menstrual cycle if you are menstruating. Other tests may include testosterone, progesterone (usually done on day twenty-one to check for ovulation), luteinizing hormone, and DHEA levels (which are checked for polycystic ovarian syndrome and/or annovulatory bleeding), and thyroid tests. In 2004, researchers even proposed that ultrasound may let doctors predict how many fertile years a woman has left by measuring the size of her ovaries! However, this test, described in the July 2004 edition of the journal *Human Reproduction*, has not yet been tested on women.

Saliva testing is often recommended by alternative medicine practitioners as a way to determine if a woman has the right balance of hormones, or if she is experiencing hormonal deficiencies. However, conventional medical experts don't consider saliva testing a proven, reliable, or accurate test, since there's no pre-established "right" level of hormones for postmenopausal women, and hormone levels may not even be related to a woman's physical comfort.

What's Normal; What's Elevated?

Follicle-stimulating hormone levels fluctuate during a woman's menstrual cycle, but normal levels range from 5mIU/mL (milli-international units per millimeter) to 30 mIU/mL for menstruating women, to 50mIU/mL to 100 mIU/mL in menopausal women. In other words, women in menopause have FSH levels up to ten times higher. But the FSH levels can vary greatly for reasons other than menopause, including if a woman is taking hormone therapy or if she has a genetic abnormality called Turner's syndrome or anorexia nervosa; other lesser-supported causes include having ovarian or adrenal cancer, starting puberty very early, or having problems with her hormone-regulating system.

Hormone Replacement Therapy (HRT)

For years, hormone replacement therapy, or HRT, was the most common treatment for menopausal symptoms such as hot flashes and decreased libido. Many women were also given HRT to reduce their risk of heart disease and osteoporosis. However, in 2002 and again in 2004, a major study called the Women's Health Initiative (WHI) revealed that the risks of HRT, including a slightly higher risk of breast cancer, heart attack, stroke, and blood clots, greatly outweighed its benefits. However, HRT is still the best way to treat hot flashes and osteoporosis; you (and your doctor) must weigh the risks and benefits according to your own symptoms and situation.

Two separate portions of the study found HRT carried significant risks. The 2002 portion of the study focused on women with a uterus who took Prempro, a combination estrogen and progestin medication: it showed the women had a 26 percent increase in breast cancer, a 41 percent increase in strokes, and a 29 percent increase in heart attacks. The second portion of the same study focused on women without a uterus who were taking Premarin, an estrogen-only medication. It found that estrogen replacement increased stroke. Both portions of the study were stopped early when it became clear that the risks outweighed the benefits.

A third study, known as the Heart Estrogen/Progestin Replacement Study (or HERS), published earlier in 2002, found HRT had no benefit on the heart.

What Does This Mean for You?

The HRT studies, while dramatic, should not preclude all women from taking HRT for their menopause symptoms. For one, HRT has proven short-term benefits for menopause. Second, the increased risk found in the studies still translates into small numbers: 8 out of 10,000 women on estrogen-progestin HRT will develop invasive breast cancer and 7 will have a heart attack. In addition, age may affect risk for some diseases. The WHI study suggests that risk for heart disease from HRT is lower if a woman takes it earlier. Women aged fifty to fifty-nine who took estrogen have fewer heart attacks and deaths from coronary heart disease than women who took a placebo. Finally, low-dose HRT may provide as much relief as higher doses.

Using HRT skin patches or an estrogen cream are other ways to modify treatment and manage risk. For example, if you are taking HRT for vaginal dryness, you may be better off with a localized estrogen cream. Similarly, if you're using HRT to increase your libido, skin patches may be a better choice than oral medications, since a report presented at the World Congress on Menopause in 2002 found that skin patches can help women achieve orgasm better because they don't have to first pass through the liver, as oral medications do.

Experts generally recommend HRT be taken in the lowest dose for no longer than two to four years.

One caveat, HRT may sensitize your body to the hormones. If you take HRT to relieve symptoms such as hot flashes, your symptoms may actually worsen if you discontinue the medications.

Other Treatments

There are alternatives to HRT. Mood symptoms, for example, can be managed with antidepressants such as Prozac or Paxil. Blood pressure and epilepsy medications may also help.

Other physical symptoms can be treated with lifestyle changes, diet, alternative medications, and over-the-counter medications. In terms of diet, avoid spicy foods, alcohol, and caffeine to minimize hot flashes, flushing and anxiety, or irritability. Incorporating soy into the diet eases symptoms related to estrogen-loss.

Physically, you'll want to dress for rapid body temperature changes by wearing layers and light clothing, exercise three to four times a week (muscle strengthening and flexibility exercises are especially good), and quit smoking.

Relaxation techniques such as yoga or meditation can also help you manage symptoms, especially hot flashes, which can come out of the blue. Acupuncture may improve symptoms, and herbal supplements such as black cohosh may also help reduce symptoms since they contain substances called phytoestrogens that are similar to estrogen. Also some women find relief with vitamin E, although there is no clinical proof that it helps.

Finally, try over-the-counter medications such as lubricants to ease vaginal dryness and increase enjoyment during intercourse.

 # Question

Are menopause-related memory problems related to estrogen loss or to stress?
A 2003 study by researchers from Rush-Presbyterian St. Luke's Medical Center, Chicago, suggest these problems have more to do with the stress of a major life transition than hormone loss. Researchers gave memory tests to 803 women between the ages of forty-two and fifty-two and found their memory skills increased rather than decreased as they had expected.

Support Groups

Your local hospital or health clinic may offer perimenopause and menopause support groups in your area. Other organizations, such as the YMCA or Planned Parenthood, may also offer support. You can also contact groups on the Internet. A Web search for "perimenopause support" or "menopause support" should bring up plenty of online discussion groups where participants offer each other support and understanding.

Other groups that provide information and resources on peri-menopause and menopause include the American College of Obstetricians and Gynecologists (*www.acog.org*), the American Menopause Foundation (*www.americanmenopause.org*), the Society for Women's Health Research (*www.womens-health.org*), the North American Menopause Society (*www.menopause.org*), Menopause-Online.com (*www.menopause-online.com*), OBGYN.net (*www.obgyn.net*), and the National Osteoporosis Foundation (*www.nof.org*).

Saying Goodbye to PMS

The good thing about PMS is that it does not last forever. Whether through menopause, or through medical and self-care therapies, it does eventually subside. However, you have a lot of influence in how PMS impacts your life as well as your family's. Take this opportunity to reduce stress and make time for yourself, to eat better, healthier foods, and to exercise. These simple solutions may dramatically reduce your symptoms, but if that's not enough, know that medical experts have learned a lot about PMS in the last twenty years and can offer relief for pain, depression, anxiety, and a host of physical PMS-related symptoms.

A Selected List of Resources

American College of Obstetricians and Gynecologists

www.acog.org

The Center for Women's Mental Health, Massachusetts General Hospital

Evaluation and treatment of psychiatric disorders associated with female reproductive function, including PMDD, pregnancy-associated mood disturbance, postpartum psychiatric illness, and perimenopausal and postmenopausal depression

www.womensmentalhealth.org

Facts for Health

Web site sponsored by the Madison Institute of Medicine offers a comprehensive overview of PMDD

www.pmdd.factsforhealth.org

The National Association for Premenstrual Syndrome

A British association for PMS

www.pms.org.uk

National Family Planning and Reproductive Health Association

Provides advocacy, education, and training for family planning and reproductive health care

www.nfprha.org

National Institutes of Health

Information on clinical trials

www.clinicaltrials.gov

National Women's Health Information Center

Federal government resource on women's health issues

www.4women.gov

The National Women's Health Hotline, PMS Access

Information and education about premenstrual syndrome

✍️*www.womenshealth.com*

OBGYN.net

Internet-based educational resource on women's health issues

✍️*www.obgyn.net*

Premenstrual Evaluation Unit
Columbia-Presbyterian Medical Center

212-305-2500 (main hospital number)

Premenstrual Syndrome Program
University of Pennsylvania, Philadelphia, PA

This program specializes in finding effective treatment for PMS through research, providing free, confidential diagnosis and possible treatment

Hotline: 800-662-4487

Phone: 215-662-3329

PMS Glossary

Acupuncture
An ancient Chinese technique of inserting thin needles at specific points on the body called meridians to control pain, improve functioning, and cure disease.

Adrenal glands
Glands located above the kidneys that produce hormones, including estrogen, progesterone, steroids, cortisol, and cortisone, and chemicals such as adrenaline, norepinephrine, and dopamine. The glands regulate many functions in the body, including heart rate, blood pressure, and stress response.

Adrenaline
A hormone produced by the adrenal glands that is released into the bloodstream in response to stress. Adrenaline stimulates the heart, blood vessels, and respiratory system. Adrenaline is also called epinephrine.

Affective symptoms
Mood or emotional responses out of sync with or inappropriate to the behavior or stimulus that prompts them. In PMS, affective symptoms include depression, anxiety, irritability, and mood swings.

Agnus castus
The scientific name for chasteberry, an herb used to treat PMS symptoms such as irritability, anxiety, bloating, breast fullness, and headache. The complete scientific name is *Vitex agnus castus*.

Aldosterone
A hormone secreted by the adrenal glands that stimulates sodium retention.

Alternative medicine
A broad category of medical treatment systems that are not recognized by conventional or standard medicine. Alternative medicine is used in place of standard treatments. Examples include traditional Chinese medicine, herbal medicine, and naturopathy.

Amygdala
An almond-shaped structure in the part of the brain that regulates emotion and triggers response to dangers. The amygdala is implicated in many psychiatric disorders.

Androgen/androgenic hormone
A hormone that produces male characteristics and the development and function of

male sexual organs. Androgenic hormones include testosterone and androsterone.

Antiolytics
Drugs used to treat anxiety symptoms, tension, and agitation.

Aromatherapy
The practice of using essential oils from flowers, herbs, and trees to promote health, relieve stress, and promote relaxation. It is an alternative practice to treat PMS.

Ayurvedic medicine
A 5,000-year-old system of holistic and preventive medicine from India. Ayurveda treats illness as an imbalance or stress in a person's life and encourages right thinking, diet, lifestyle, and herbs.

Bipolar disorder
A mood disorder characterized by severe and often rapid alteration in mood, in which a person experiences recurrent bouts of depression alternating with mania or euphoria. It was formerly known as manic-depressive disorder.

Chiropractic
A system of treating musculoskeletal disorders by adjusting the spinal column.

Cognitive-behavioral therapy
A type of psychotherapy in which a person is taught to recognize distorted thinking and replace it with more realistic thoughts and beliefs. It is used to treat depression, anxiety disorders, phobias, and other mental illnesses.

Cognitive symptoms
Responses that affect a person's ability to perceive, think, and remember. In PMS, these might include difficulty concentrating and memory problems.

Complementary medicine
Noninvasive, nonpharmaceutical medical techniques used to treat illness and disease. These techniques are used in conjunction with more conventional medical treatments, such as drug therapy and surgery. Examples of complementary medicine practices include dietary supplements, herbal medicine, meditation, and acupuncture.

Corpus luteum
A structure formed in the ovary from the cells that remain after an egg has been released. The corpus luteum produces progesterone to support a woman's pregnancy and prevent menstruation.

Cortisol
A steroid hormone produced by the adrenal glands in response to stress. It is important in maintaining blood insulin levels, body fluids, and electrolytes.

Cyclothymia
A chronic bipolar disorder with short periods of mild depression and hypomania (which consists of elevated mood, irritability, optimism, a decreased need for sleep, and increased talkativeness). Some people with this disorder go on to develop full-blown bipolar disorder.

Diuretics
Drugs that increase the production and excretion of urine. They are used to remove fluid from the body and reduce bloating.

Dopamine

A neurotransmitter critical to muscle movement, insulin regulation, physical energy, thinking, short-term memory, and emotion.

Dysmenorrhea

Pain or discomfort before or during menstrual periods. Primary dysmenorrhea is pain that does not have a separate medical cause; secondary dysmenorrhea is pain that is caused by a condition other than menstruation, such as endometriosis.

Dysthymic disorder

Depression characterized by a lack of enjoyment or pleasure in life that continues for at least two years.

Electrolytes

Minerals that regulate bodily functions, including the body's fluid balance and muscle contraction. Electrolytes include potassium, calcium, chloride, bicarbonate, and magnesium.

Endocrine

Having to do with hormones and the glands that produce and secrete them in the body.

Endometriosis

A condition in which endometrial tissue, which lines the uterine cavity, grows in locations outside the uterus, such as the ovaries, fallopian tubes, and abdominal cavity. It is a painful condition that causes heavy bleeding and scarring and may lead to infertility.

Endorphins

Opium-like chemicals naturally produced by the brain that elevate mood and kill pain.

Estradiol

The main hormone produced by the follicular cells of the ovary.

Estriol

A weak estrogen hormone that increases during pregnancy.

Estrogen

A primary sex hormone produced by the ovaries, placenta, and adrenal glands. Estrogen is responsible for the development of female sex characteristics.

Estrone

An estrogenic hormone produced by the ovarian follicles. It is weaker than estradiol.

Evening primrose oil

A nutritional supplement made from a weedy plant that contains essential fatty acids, especially gamma-linolenic acid. It is used to relieve pain and inflammation. In PMS, it has been found helpful in reducing breast tenderness.

Fibrocystic breast condition

A condition in which there is fibrous tissue in the breasts; the condition of having lumpy breasts.

Fibromyalgia

A chronic disorder characterized by widespread musculoskeletal pain, fatigue, soft-tissue tenderness, and sleep disorder.

Fluoxetine

A selective serotonin reuptake inhibitor used to treat depression and premenstrual dysphoric disorder. Brand names include Prozac and Sarafem.

Follicular phase
The first phase of the menstrual cycle during which the egg follicles in the ovaries grow and endometrial tissue in the uterus thickens.

FSH-RF
Follicle-stimulating hormone-releasing factor; a chemical secreted by the pituitary gland that prompts the body to release follicle-stimulating hormone.

Homeopathy
The medical practice of treating disease by using very small doses of substances that in a healthy person would produce symptoms similar to the disease.

Hyperhydration
Water intoxication, in which a person's intake of water is excessive. In PMS, hyperhydration refers to fluid retention, weight gain, breast tenderness, and swelling of the extremities.

Hypoadrenia
A term used by alternative medicine to describe a reduction in adrenal activity. This condition is not recognized by conventional medicine.

Hypoglycemia
Abnormally low blood sugar. It can cause jitteriness, rapid breathing, and lethargy.

Hypomania
A mild form of mania.

Hypothalamus
A small structure at the base of the brain that regulates the endocrine process, body temperature, sleep, and appetite.

Hypothyroidism
A condition of having too little thyroid hormone, which leads to a lowered metabolic rate, weight gain, and a loss of energy. This condition is also known as underactive thyroid.

Hysterectomy
The surgical removal of the uterus and sometimes the cervix.

GABA
Gamma-aminobutyric acid is the primary neurotransmitter in the brain. It is involved in muscle relaxation, diminished emotional reaction, and sedation.

Generalized anxiety disorder
An anxiety disorder in which a person has excessive and uncontrollable anxiety for six months or longer, often without apparent cause.

Gonadotropin
A hormone that stimulates the gonads (ovaries in women, testes in men).

GnRH agonists
A group of drugs that suppress the pituitary gland in order to suppress the ovaries. GnRH agonists induce menopause-like symptoms and are commonly used to treat endometriosis.

Leptin
A hormone that helps regulate a person's appetite and metabolism.

Light therapy
A treatment that uses very bright full-spectrum light for a prescribed amount of time to promote a normal sleep-wake

cycle and decrease sleep disturbances. It is used to treat seasonal affective disorder. It is also known as phototherapy.

Luteal phase
The second half of the menstrual cycle during which an egg becomes a corpus luteum and produces progesterone.

Luteinizing hormone
A hormone produced by the pituitary gland that stimulates ovulation.

Mania
A medical condition characterized by severely elevated mood.

Mastalgia
Pain in the breast; the condition of painful breasts.

Melatonin
A hormone produced by the pineal gland in the brain in response to darkness. It regulates the onset and timing of sleep rhythms.

Menopause
The stage in life when a woman stops having menstrual periods. On average, this happens at age fifty-two.

Menstrual migraine
A type of migraine headache that occurs only during menstruation or at ovulation.

Mood lability
The quality of unstable or quickly changing moods.

Myomectomy
The surgical removal of fibroids. The procedure leaves the uterus intact.

Naturopathy
A holistic system of medicine originating in Europe that uses natural substances to balance a person's internal chemistry. Naturopathy avoids drugs and surgery and instead relies on nutrition, herbal medicine, and homeopathy.

Neurohormones
Biochemical substances made by tissues in the body that stimulate the cells to which they attach.

Neuropsychiatrist
A physician concerned with the study of the brain and mental diseases.

Neurotransmitters
Chemical substances that carry impulses from one nerve cell to another. They include serotonin, norepinephrine, and acetylcholine.

Norepinephrine
A neurotransmitter and hormone involved in the body's fight-or-flight response to stress; it is involved in alertness, concentration, aggression, motivation.

NSAIDs
Nonsteroidal anti-inflammatory drugs; a group of drugs used to relive pain, fever, and inflammation, such as aspirin, ibuprofen, and naproxen.

Oophorectomy
Surgery to remove one or both ovaries. This is a last-resort treatment for PMS since it causes premature menopause.

Ovulation
The release of a mature egg from an ovary.

Ovulatory phase
The phase of a menstrual cycle when ovulation occurs (generally, but not necessarily, the midpoint of the menstrual cycle).

Perimenopause
The transition period before menopause. Symptoms include decreased production of estrogen and progesterone, irregular menstrual periods, hot flashes, and night sweats, as well as mood changes.

Pilates
An exercise technique based on the work of Joseph Pilates designed to strengthen core muscles, increase flexibility, and improve posture.

Placebo
An inactive substance that has no treatment value. It is used in clinical trials as a control to evaluate the effectiveness of experimental treatment.

Postpartum depression
Depression that occurs after childbirth.

Precursor
A substance from which another substance is formed. For example, tryptophan is a precursor to serotonin, which means it is the source of serotonin.

Premenstrual dysphoric disorder
PMDD; a severe form of premenstrual syndrome characterized by severe depression, shifting moods, difficulty concentrating, irritability, anxiety, and tension, as well as physical symptoms such as bloating, headache, and joint and muscle pain.

Premenstrual magnification
The worsening of certain illnesses and symptoms during the premenstrual phase.

Progesterone
A female steroid hormone secreted by the ovary. It prepares the uterus for the fertilized ovum and maintains the pregnancy. Synthetic progesterone is used in oral contraceptives.

Progestin
The synthetic form of progesterone.

Prolactin
A hormone produced by the pituitary gland that stimulates breast development and milk production.

Prostaglandins
Hormone-like substances produced in the uterus that control inflammation, control contractions, and may cause cramps.

Psychological symptoms
Symptoms of PMS that affect both mood and cognition. Examples include depression, confusion, and forgetfulness.

Psychotherapy
Types of treatment that involve talking and listening, usually with a psychiatrist, psychologist, social worker, or licensed counselor.

Randomized controlled trial
Clinical trial in which study participants are assigned randomly either an intervention being tested or a placebo. Randomized controlled trials are highly reliable because the study design avoids bias.

Reflexology
A form of massage in which pressure is applied to specific areas on the feet, hands, and ears to promote health and relaxation.

Sarafem
The brand name of the SSRI fluoxetine hydrochloride; used to treat premenstrual dysphoric disorder.

Schizoaffective disorder
A mental disorder in which the person exhibits both mood symptoms and psychosis, such as hallucinations and delusions.

Seasonal affective disorder
A mood disorder that is related to the change of seasons, developing in the winter when sunlight is limited and resolving in the spring.

Selective serotonin reuptake inhibitors
SSRIs; antidepressant drugs that selectively inhibit the absorption of serotonin at certain nerve membranes. SSRIs make the brain use serotonin more efficiently.

Serotonin
A neurotransmitter that affects behavior, emotions, and thought, serotonin also causes blood vessels to narrow. It is involved in mood disorders, such as depression and PMDD. Serotonin is also known as 5-hydroxytryptamine.

Somatic
Having to do with the body. Somatic PMS symptoms include muscle and joint pain, headaches, and so on.

Soy isoflavones
Nutrients isolated from soybeans, isoflavones include genistein and daidzein. They are thought to be very beneficial for PMS.

Testosterone
The male sex hormone, it promotes the development of male characteristics. Women have small amounts of testosterone in their bodies.

Thyroid disease
An abnormality of the thyroid gland and its production of thyroid hormone.

Tricyclic antidepressants
A class of medications used to treat depression; named after the drugs' molecular structure, which contains three rings of atoms. SSRIs largely replaced TCAs as the preferred treatment for depressive disorders.

Triphasic oral contraceptives
Oral contraceptives in which the ratio of estrogen and progestin varies in three phases over the course of the cycle. This pattern more closely mimics a woman's natural menstrual cycle.

Tryptophan
An essential amino acid formed from proteins during digestion. It is essential for normal growth and development and is a precursor to serotonin.

Weight cycling
Rapidly losing and then regaining weight, also known as yo-yo dieting.

Index